I0844472

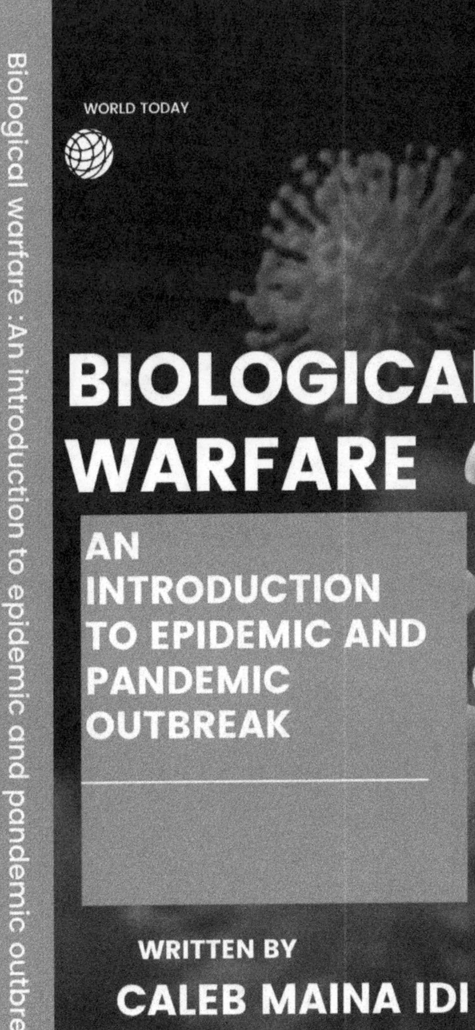

WORLD TODAY
2023 EDITION
BIOLOGICAL WARFARE
AN INTRODUCTION TO EPIDEMIC AND PANDEMIC OUTBREAK
WRITTEN BY
CALEB MAINA IDI

Biological warfare :An introduction to epidemic and pandemic outbrea

BIOLOGICAL WARFARE

An introduction to Epidemic and Pandemic Outbreak

CALEB MAINA IDI

Table of Contents

Preface

Introduction

- Defining Biological Warfare
- Historical Overview of Biological Warfare
- The Scope of Epidemic and Pandemic Outbreaks

Part I: The Science of Biological Warfare

1. Understanding Pathogens
- Bacteria, Viruses, and Toxins
- Weaponization of Biological Agents
2. The Lethal Potential
- Biological Agents and Their Effects
- Mechanisms of Infection and Transmission

Part II: Historical Perspectives
3. Ancient and Medieval Biological Warfare

- Early Instances of Bioweapons
- The Use of Plague as a Weapon

4. 20th Century Biowarfare Programs
- World War I and World War II
- Cold War Bioweapons Programs

Part III: Modern Bioweapon Threats
5. State-Sponsored Biological Warfare

- Notable Offenders
- International Agreements and Treaties

6. Non-State Actors and Terrorism
- Bioterrorism and its Threats
- Case Studies and Incidents

Part IV: The Science of Epidemics and Pandemics

Preface

In an increasingly interconnected world, the specter of biological warfare looms as a dark shadow over humanity. The potential for the malicious use of biological agents to incite epidemic and pandemic outbreaks is a topic of paramount importance. This book, "Biological Warfare: An Introduction to Epidemic and Pandemic Outbreak," delves into the ominous realm where science, security, and the fragility of our species converge.

The pages that follow will navigate the intricate web of biological weapons, the insidious pathogens that can be harnessed, and the perilous consequences that may unfold. From the early history of biowarfare to contemporary global threats, this book aims to be a comprehensive primer, offering insights into the science, politics, and ethics surrounding biological warfare.

In a world still grappling with the aftermath of recent pandemics, the urgency of understanding the intricacies of biological warfare cannot be overstated. This book is not just a chronicle of peril but a call to action. It seeks to empower readers with knowledge, stimulate discourse, and foster a collective commitment to safeguarding our species from this most insidious form of warfare.

As we embark on this journey through the shadowy realm of biological warfare, let us remain vigilant, informed, and united in our determination to prevent, mitigate, and respond to the threats that loom on the horizon. The battle for our biological security begins with knowledge, and this book aims to provide a foundational understanding of a topic that, though chilling, demands our unwavering attention.

Together, let us embark on this exploration of the clandestine world of biological warfare, for in knowledge lies our greatest defense against the darkness that threatens our collective well-being.

Caleb Maina Idi
26th August 2023

Introduction

Biological Warfare: An Introduction to Epidemic and Pandemic Outbreaks

In the annals of human history, warfare has taken on many forms - from ancient battles waged with swords and shields to modern conflicts characterized by advanced weaponry and technology. Yet, among the myriad strategies employed in the theater of war, one method has struck terror into the hearts of nations for centuries: biological warfare.

Biological warfare, or biowarfare, refers to the deliberate use of pathogens - bacteria, viruses, fungi, or toxins - as weapons to incapacitate or kill an adversary. It is a form of warfare that extends far beyond traditional military engagements, infiltrating the very essence of life itself. In recent years, the world has been confronted with the stark reality that the boundaries between natural pandemics and biowarfare-induced outbreaks are becoming increasingly blurred.

The Historical Precursors

The notion of using disease as a weapon is not a recent development. Throughout history, there have been unsettling instances where pathogens have been weaponized, often with devastating consequences. The most infamous example can be traced back to antiquity when besieging armies would hurl corpses infected with deadly diseases over city walls, leading to the outbreak of epidemics within the besieged walls. Such crude tactics were the earliest forms of biological warfare.

One of the earliest recorded instances of biological warfare occurred during the Peloponnesian War (431-404 BC), when the city-state of Athens fell victim to a mysterious plague. Historical accounts, notably Thucydides' writings, describe symptoms resembling those of typhoid fever or Ebola. The cause of this plague remains a subject of speculation, but many historians believe it to be one of the earliest documented instances of biowarfare. It is suspected that the Spartans deliberately contaminated the Athenians' water supply with disease, leading to the catastrophic outbreak.

The Modern Era of Biological Warfare

The 20th century ushered in a new era of biowarfare, characterized by scientific advancements and an alarming escalation of potential threats. World War I witnessed the deployment of poison gas as a battlefield weapon, foreshadowing the dark possibilities of manipulating biological agents for destructive purposes.

The horrific events of World War II saw the intensification of biological warfare research by several nations, most notably Nazi Germany and Imperial Japan. Notorious figures such as Dr. Shiro Ishii and his Unit 731 conducted inhumane experiments on prisoners of war, exploring the weaponization of biological agents like anthrax and the bubonic plague. These actions revealed the depths to which humans could descend in their quest for destructive power.

As World War II drew to a close, the international community recognized the urgent need to address the threat posed by biological warfare. The Biological Weapons Convention (BWC) of 1972 emerged as a pivotal milestone, with over 180 nations agreeing to renounce the development, production, and stockpiling of biological weapons. However, the specter of biowarfare never truly vanished; instead, it evolved in the shadowy realm of covert research programs and state-sponsored terrorism.

The Dual-Use Dilemma

One of the gravest challenges posed by biological warfare lies in its dual-use nature. Unlike nuclear weapons, which have limited civilian applications, biological agents have numerous legitimate uses in medicine, agriculture, and biotechnology. This duality makes it exceptionally challenging to monitor and control research and development activities, as the very knowledge and infrastructure necessary for beneficial purposes can also be harnessed for destructive ones.

Scientific progress has, paradoxically, both enabled our ability to combat infectious diseases and enhanced our capacity for biowarfare. Advances in genetic engineering and synthetic biology, for instance, have unlocked the potential to design custom pathogens with specific properties, such as increased virulence or antibiotic resistance. While these breakthroughs hold promise for developing vaccines and treatments, they also offer new avenues for the creation of bioengineered weapons.

The Emergence of Natural and Synthetic Pandemics

The world has been jolted into a new awareness of the devastating consequences of infectious diseases through events such as the HIV/AIDS pandemic in the late 20th century and, more recently, the COVID-19 pandemic. While these pandemics are primarily attributed to natural processes, the lines between natural and synthetic pandemics have become increasingly blurred.

The COVID-19 pandemic serves as a stark reminder of how a naturally occurring virus can rapidly spread across the globe, overwhelming healthcare systems and causing immense social and economic disruptions. However, conspiracy theories and concerns about the origins of the virus have sparked debates about the possibility of accidental or intentional release from a laboratory setting, highlighting the uneasy intersection between scientific research and biowarfare concerns.

The Unsettling Future

In our interconnected world, where pathogens can traverse borders with ease, the threat of biological warfare looms larger than ever before. As we delve deeper into the 21st century, new challenges arise. Climate change, urbanization, and increasing global mobility create fertile ground for the emergence and spread of infectious diseases, whether through natural processes or malevolent intent.

In this era, where information spreads as rapidly as viruses, vigilance and preparedness are our greatest allies. The realm of biological warfare is no longer confined to military bunkers; it extends to laboratories, cyberspace, and the very ecosystems we depend upon. Understanding the intricate web that connects biological warfare, epidemics, and pandemics is essential for safeguarding our future.

In the pages that follow, we will delve deeper into the history, science, and ethical dimensions of biological warfare. We will explore the mechanisms by which pathogens can be weaponized, the international efforts to prevent biowarfare, and the ethical dilemmas that arise in our quest for knowledge and security. This exploration is not merely an academic exercise but a call to vigilance, urging us to navigate the delicate balance between scientific progress and the preservation of our collective safety.

As we embark on this journey into the heart of biological warfare and its connection to epidemic and pandemic outbreaks, let us not forget the lessons of history and the imperatives of our time. The future of our world may well hinge on our ability to confront the complexities of this dark and perilous domain.

Defining Biological Warfare: A Comprehensive Examination

Introduction

Biological warfare, often referred to as biowarfare or germ warfare, is a form of warfare that employs biological agents, such as bacteria, viruses, toxins, and fungi, with the intent to harm or kill humans, animals, or plants. This form of warfare is as old as recorded history, with instances dating back to ancient times when attackers used various biological agents to weaken their adversaries. Over the centuries, the methods and consequences of biological warfare have evolved significantly, making it a topic of great concern in the modern world.

This essay aims to define biological warfare comprehensively by examining its history, the types of biological agents employed, the methods of dissemination, its impacts on society, international efforts to control it, and the ethical considerations surrounding its use.

Historical Perspective

Ancient and Medieval Use

The use of biological agents as weapons can be traced back thousands of years. Historical records suggest that in ancient times, besiegers would hurl corpses or animal carcasses over the walls of fortified cities to spread disease among the inhabitants. The bodies acted as vectors for various pathogens, including bacteria and viruses, which would lead to outbreaks of deadly diseases within the city walls. These crude methods demonstrated an early understanding of the potential of biological agents as weapons.

One notable example is the Siege of Caffa in 1347-1348 during the Black Death pandemic. According to accounts, Mongol attackers catapulted plague-infected corpses into the city, leading to the outbreak of the bubonic plague among the defenders. This early form of biological warfare showcased the devastating consequences of using disease as a weapon.

Modern Era and World War I

Biological warfare continued to be a threat in the modern era. During World War I, several nations, including Germany, the United Kingdom, and the United States, conducted research into the use of biological agents as weapons. However, these efforts did not result in widespread use during the conflict.

Types of Biological Agents

Biological agents used in warfare can be classified into several categories:

Bacteria

Bacterial agents include pathogens such as anthrax (Bacillus anthracis), plague (Yersinia pestis), and tularemia (Francisella tularensis). These bacteria can be weaponized in various forms, such as spores or aerosols, to infect humans or animals.

Anthrax is particularly notorious due to its resilience as spores can survive in the environment for extended periods. In 2001, the United States experienced a bioterrorism attack when anthrax spores were sent through the mail, resulting in several deaths and widespread fear.

Viruses

Viruses used in biological warfare include smallpox, Ebola, and Marburg virus. Smallpox, caused by the variola virus, was one of the deadliest diseases in history and was eradicated through vaccination efforts. However, concerns exist regarding the potential existence of smallpox stocks in clandestine laboratories or bioweapons programs.

Toxins

Toxins, such as ricin and botulinum toxin, are produced by living organisms and can be extracted and weaponized. These toxins can be lethal in small quantities and can be disseminated through various means, including aerosols and contamination of food or water supplies.

Fungi

Fungi like Aspergillus flavus and Aflatoxin-producing species can be used as biological agents. They are capable of producing mycotoxins, which can contaminate food crops and cause serious health issues when ingested.

Dissemination Methods

Biological agents can be disseminated in several ways, each with its own advantages and challenges:

Aerosols

Aerosol dissemination involves converting the biological agent into tiny particles suspended in the air. This method allows for the efficient spread of pathogens over a wide area. However, it requires specialized equipment and poses risks to the attackers themselves, as they can also be exposed to the agents.

Contamination

Contamination methods involve introducing biological agents into water supplies, food sources, or the environment. This can lead to the slow, indirect exposure of the targeted population. Contamination methods are less immediate but can be difficult to trace back to the attacker.

Direct Transmission

Direct transmission involves infecting individuals or animals and using them as carriers to spread the disease. This method is often less controlled and predictable than other methods.

Impacts on Society

The use of biological warfare can have profound and far-reaching impacts on society:

Health Consequences

The immediate consequence of a biological attack is a public health crisis. Diseases can spread rapidly, overwhelming healthcare systems and causing high mortality rates. In addition to death and illness, survivors may experience long-term health effects, and the psychological toll can be immense.

Economic Disruption

Biological attacks can disrupt economies by causing illness, death, and fear, leading to decreased productivity and increased healthcare costs. Agricultural-based biological attacks can also devastate food supplies, leading to food shortages and economic instability.

Societal Disruption

The fear and panic resulting from a biological attack can lead to social upheaval. Quarantines, travel restrictions, and loss of trust in institutions can erode social cohesion and stability.

Environmental Consequences

Biological agents can have unintended environmental impacts. For example, the introduction of pathogens or toxins into ecosystems can harm wildlife and disrupt delicate ecological balances.

International Efforts to Control Biological Warfare

The international community has recognized the grave threat posed by biological warfare and has taken steps to control its use:

Biological Weapons Convention (BWC)

The Biological Weapons Convention, established in 1972, is an international treaty that prohibits the development, production, and acquisition of biological weapons. It also mandates the destruction of existing stockpiles. While the BWC has been successful in curbing the overt development of biological weapons, challenges remain in verifying compliance and preventing covert programs.

United Nations Security Council Resolutions

The United Nations Security Council has passed resolutions aimed at strengthening global efforts to combat biological warfare. These resolutions emphasize the need for robust and effective measures to prevent the proliferation of biological weapons.

Global Health Security Agenda (GHSA)

The GHSA is an international partnership that focuses on strengthening health systems and response capabilities to prevent, detect, and respond to biological threats, including natural outbreaks and bioterrorism.

Ethical Considerations

The use of biological warfare raises profound ethical questions:

Humanitarian Principles

The use of biological agents as weapons violates fundamental humanitarian principles, including the principle of proportionality and the distinction between combatants and civilians. Biological attacks often result in indiscriminate harm to innocent civilians.

Accountability

Identifying the perpetrators of a biological attack can be challenging. This lack of accountability can embolden state and non-state actors to use biological weapons with relative impunity.

Dual-Use Dilemma

The dual-use nature of biotechnology and the life sciences presents a dilemma. Advances in these fields have the potential to benefit humanity, but they can also be exploited for malevolent purposes. Striking a balance between scientific progress and security is a complex challenge.

Biological warfare, with its devastating potential for harm, poses a significant threat to humanity. Understanding the historical context, types of biological agents, methods of dissemination, and societal impacts is crucial for addressing this threat effectively. International efforts, such as the Biological Weapons Convention and the Global Health Security Agenda, play a vital role in preventing war.

Historical Overview of Biological Warfare

Biological warfare, the use of biological agents to harm or kill humans, animals, or plants, has a long and dark history. This form of warfare predates the modern era and has evolved significantly over time. This overview will examine the historical development of biological warfare, exploring its origins, major events, key players, and the ethical dilemmas it presents.

Ancient Origins (Pre-20th Century)

1.   Early Uses of Biological Warfare: The concept of using disease as a weapon can be traced back to ancient times, with examples such as the use of infected animal carcasses during sieges in antiquity.
2.   Bioterrorism in Ancient India: The use of poisonous snakes and toxins in warfare is documented in ancient Indian texts like the "Arthashastra."

Biological Warfare in the Modern Era (20th Century)

1.   World War I: The use of chemical and biological agents during WWI, including chlorine gas and anthrax, marked the modern era of biological warfare.
2.   Interwar Period: Efforts to ban biological weapons through international treaties like the Geneva Protocol of 1925 were largely unsuccessful.
3.   World War II: Japan's infamous Unit 731 conducted inhumane experiments with biological agents on prisoners of war, leading to significant advancements in biowarfare.

The Cold War Era

1.   Biological Arms Race: The Cold War saw both the United States and the Soviet Union develop extensive biowarfare programs, stockpiling dangerous pathogens.
2.   Biological Weapons Convention (BWC) of 1972: The BWC aimed to prohibit the development, production, and acquisition of biological weapons, but enforcement remained challenging.

Post-Cold War Developments

1.   Iraq's Bioweapons Program: Saddam Hussein's Iraq pursued biological weapons, which were a concern during the Gulf War and its aftermath.

2.   Aum Shinrikyo: The Japanese cult Aum Shinrikyo attempted to use anthrax in terrorist attacks in the 1990s.

Modern Concerns

1.   Biological Terrorism: In the 21st century, there is a growing concern about the potential use of biological agents by terrorists.
2.   Dual-Use Research: Advances in biotechnology raise ethical dilemmas, as research can have both peaceful and harmful applications.

International Efforts and Ethical Considerations

1.   Biological Weapons Convention (BWC) in the 21st Century: Efforts to strengthen the BWC and improve compliance with its provisions.
2.   Ethical Dilemmas: The ethical challenges of biowarfare, including the risk of accidental release, the difficulty of attribution, and the potential for mass casualties.

The history of biological warfare is a troubling one, marked by instances of ruthless experimentation and the potential for widespread devastation. Efforts to control and prohibit biological weapons continue to be a critical component of international security. As technology advances, the ethical and practical challenges of preventing the use of biological agents in warfare remain a pressing concern for the global community.

The Scope of Epidemic and Pandemic Outbreaks

Epidemic and pandemic outbreaks have been an integral part of human history, shaping societies and civilizations in profound ways. From the Black Death in the 14th century to the COVID-19 pandemic that began in 2019, these events have demonstrated the remarkable capacity of infectious diseases to disrupt and transform the world. This essay explores the scope of epidemic and pandemic outbreaks, delving into their causes, impacts, responses, and the lessons they offer for the future.

I. The Basics of Epidemics and Pandemics

1.1 Definitions

To begin, it is essential to clarify the terms 'epidemic' and 'pandemic':

•	Epidemic: An epidemic is the rapid spread of an infectious disease to a large number of people within a specific geographic area or community. The key characteristic is an unusually high number of cases compared to what is normally expected.
•	Pandemic: A pandemic is a global outbreak of an infectious disease, often caused by a novel pathogen to which a large portion of the population has little or no immunity. Pandemics involve sustained human-to-human transmission across multiple countries or continents.

1.2 Causes of Epidemics and Pandemics

Epidemics and pandemics arise from a combination of factors, including:

1.2.1 Pathogens: The microorganisms responsible for these outbreaks are diverse, including bacteria, viruses, fungi, and parasites. Their ability to adapt and mutate can enhance their virulence and transmissibility.

1.2.2 Host Factors: Population density, age, health status, and vaccination rates all affect how readily an infectious disease spreads within a community.

1.2.3 Environmental Factors: Climate, sanitation, and living conditions play a significant role in the transmission of diseases. For example, some pathogens thrive in warm and humid environments, while others are more stable in cold and dry conditions.

1.2.4 Globalization: Increased travel and trade have facilitated the rapid spread of infectious diseases. A disease that once might have been confined to a single village can now traverse the globe within days.

II. Historical Examples of Epidemics and Pandemics

2.1 The Black Death (1347-1351)

One of the most infamous pandemics in history, the Black Death, was caused by the bacterium Yersinia pestis. It swept through Europe, Asia, and Africa, claiming an estimated 75-200 million lives. This pandemic had a profound impact on medieval society, leading to labor shortages and significant changes in economic and social structures.

2.2 The Spanish Flu (1918-1919)

The Spanish flu, caused by an H1N1 influenza virus, remains one of the deadliest pandemics in modern history. It infected one-third of the global population and caused an estimated 50 million deaths. The rapid global movement of troops during World War I played a crucial role in its spread.

2.3 HIV/AIDS Pandemic (1980s-present)

HIV/AIDS, caused by the human immunodeficiency virus (HIV), was first identified in the 1980s. It has since infected more than 75 million people worldwide, with over 32 million deaths. This pandemic has had a lasting impact on public health and has spurred significant research and advocacy efforts.

2.4 COVID-19 Pandemic (2019-present)

The COVID-19 pandemic, caused by the novel coronavirus SARS-CoV-2, began in Wuhan, China, in late 2019 and quickly spread globally. It has led to over 200 million confirmed cases and more than 4 million deaths worldwide. The pandemic has disrupted economies, strained healthcare systems, and prompted unprecedented vaccination campaigns.

III. The Impact of Epidemics and Pandemics

3.1 Public Health

Epidemics and pandemics strain healthcare systems and resources. They often lead to overwhelmed hospitals, shortages of medical supplies, and the need for rapid response strategies.

3.2 Social and Economic Impact

The economic consequences of epidemics and pandemics can be severe. Lockdowns, travel restrictions, and business closures have led to job losses, economic recessions, and increased poverty rates.

3.3 Psychological Effects

Fear and anxiety accompany outbreaks. Stigmatization of affected individuals and communities can exacerbate mental health issues. Quarantine measures, while necessary, can lead to isolation and loneliness.

3.4 Disruption of Daily Life

School closures, canceled events, and restrictions on gatherings disrupt daily routines. People may face difficulties accessing essential services and supplies.

IV. Responding to Epidemics and Pandemics

4.1 Surveillance and Early Detection

Early detection is vital for controlling epidemics. Surveillance systems, both local and global, monitor disease trends and provide data for rapid response.

4.2 Vaccination

Vaccination is one of the most effective tools for preventing epidemics and pandemics. The development of vaccines against diseases like polio, smallpox, and now COVID-19 has saved countless lives.

4.3 Public Health Measures

Non-pharmaceutical interventions such as social distancing, mask-wearing, and quarantine measures can slow the spread of infectious diseases, buying time for vaccine development and distribution.

4.4 International Cooperation

Global collaboration is essential during pandemics. Sharing information, resources, and expertise can help control the spread of diseases across borders.

V. Lessons Learned and Future Preparedness

5.1 Lessons from History

Historical pandemics have taught us the importance of early detection, swift response, and equitable access to healthcare resources.

5.2 The Role of Science and Technology

Advancements in science and technology, such as genomics and data analytics, have enabled more rapid vaccine development and improved tracking of disease spread.

5.3 Vaccine Equity

Ensuring equitable access to vaccines is crucial for global health security. Vaccine nationalism and hoarding can prolong pandemics.

5.4 Strengthening Healthcare Systems

Investing in healthcare infrastructure and workforce training can improve a country's ability to respond to epidemics.

5.5 Behavioral and Cultural Factors

Understanding cultural norms and behaviors is critical for effective public health messaging during outbreaks.

Epidemic and pandemic outbreaks are recurring events in human history. They are shaped by a complex interplay of pathogens, host factors, and environmental conditions. The historical impact of these events is profound, from reshaping societies to influencing economies and healthcare systems.

Effective responses to epidemics and pandemics require early detection, international cooperation, and equitable access to healthcare resources. Lessons learned from past outbreaks, advances in science and technology, and a commitment to strengthening healthcare systems are all essential for future preparedness.

As we move forward, it is crucial to remember that epidemics and pandemics are not isolated events but part of an ongoing dynamic. By applying the knowledge gained from past experiences, we can better navigate the challenges they present and work toward a healthier and more resilient global community.

Part I: The Science of Biological Warfare

The concept of biological warfare, the use of infectious agents as weapons, has been a source of fear and fascination for centuries. In the annals of warfare, the use of pathogens to incapacitate or kill enemy combatants is not a recent development. What has evolved over time, however, is our understanding of the science behind biological warfare and the potential consequences it holds for humanity.

This essay will delve into the science of biological warfare, exploring its history, the microorganisms and toxins involved, methods of dissemination, and the challenges it poses in the modern world. It is important to recognize that this topic, while fascinating, is fraught with ethical and moral concerns. The discussion here is intended to be purely informative, with no intent to encourage or promote harmful activities.

Historical Perspective

Biological warfare, sometimes referred to as biowarfare, has deep historical roots. The use of infectious agents as weapons can be traced back to ancient times, with instances of contaminated water sources and animal carcasses being used to spread disease among enemies. One infamous example is the siege of Caffa in 1347, during which Mongol forces catapulted plague-ridden corpses over the city walls, leading to the outbreak of the Black Death within the city.

In more recent history, biological warfare took a more organized and systematic form during World War I and World War II. Various nations, including the United States and the Soviet Union, conducted research into the development of bioweapons. The Japanese Unit 731 during World War II conducted inhumane experiments with biological agents on prisoners of war.

The Biological Weapons Convention (BWC) of 1972, which currently has 183 member states, sought to prohibit the development, production, and stockpiling of biological weapons. However, concerns about compliance and verification persist to this day.

Microorganisms and Toxins

Biological warfare agents can be categorized into several classes, including bacteria, viruses, toxins, and fungi. Each of these classes presents its own unique challenges and threats.

1.   Bacteria: Bacterial agents, such as anthrax (Bacillus anthracis) and plague (Yersinia pestis), have been of significant concern in biowarfare due to their ability to cause disease in humans and animals. These agents can be engineered for increased virulence and resistance to antibiotics.

2.   Viruses: Viral agents like smallpox (Variola virus) and Ebola (Ebola virus) have the potential for devastating outbreaks if used as bioweapons. They are highly infectious and can spread rapidly, causing widespread illness and death.

3.   Toxins: Toxins produced by certain bacteria and fungi, such as botulinum toxin and ricin, are exceptionally lethal even in small quantities. These toxins can be disseminated through various means, including aerosols, food, or contaminated water.

4.   Fungi: While less commonly discussed, fungal agents like Coccidioides spp. and Aspergillus spp. can cause severe respiratory illnesses and pose a risk in biowarfare scenarios.

Methods of Dissemination

The effectiveness of biological warfare agents often hinges on the methods used to disseminate them. There are several means by which these agents can be spread, each with its own implications.

1.   Aerosolization: Aerosolizing pathogens allows for their distribution over large areas through the air. This method can lead to respiratory infections in exposed individuals and can cause widespread outbreaks.

2.   Contaminated Food and Water: Agents can be introduced into food or water supplies, leading to ingestion and subsequent infection of those who consume them.

3.   Animal Vectors: In some cases, agents can be introduced into animal populations, leading to zoonotic transmission to humans. This method can be difficult to control and predict.

4.   Direct Contact: Direct transmission of pathogens through physical contact with contaminated individuals or surfaces is also possible. This method may be less effective for widespread dissemination but can still cause localized outbreaks.

5.   Covert Delivery: Modern advancements in biotechnology have raised concerns about the potential for covert delivery of biological agents. This could involve the modification of common microbes to carry a payload of harmful genes or toxins.

Challenges in Modern Biological Warfare

Advancements in science and technology have both expanded our understanding of biological agents and increased the potential for their misuse. Several key challenges are posed by modern biological warfare:

1.   Dual-Use Research: Many scientific advancements can be applied both for beneficial purposes and for malicious intent. Dual-use research, such as gene editing techniques like CRISPR-Cas9, can potentially be used to enhance the virulence or resistance of bioweapons.

2.   Synthetic Biology: The field of synthetic biology enables the design and creation of biological organisms or agents from scratch. This technology has the potential to create entirely new threats that may not exist in nature.

3.   Rapid Global Travel: Modern transportation systems allow infectious agents to be spread quickly across the globe. This raises concerns about the potential for bioweapons to cause pandemics.

4.   Attribution Challenges: Determining the source of a biological attack can be exceedingly difficult, as natural outbreaks and intentional releases can appear very similar. This makes it challenging to attribute an event to an act of bioterrorism.

5.   Ethics and Morality: The ethical dilemmas surrounding biological warfare are profound. Deliberate harm to civilians and non-combatants is widely condemned, and the use of bioweapons raises significant moral questions.

International Efforts and Regulations

Despite the challenges posed by biological warfare, there have been significant international efforts to prevent its use. The Biological Weapons Convention (BWC), as mentioned earlier, has played a central role in regulating the development and use of bioweapons. Additionally, organizations like the World Health Organization (WHO) and the Centers for Disease Control and Prevention (CDC) are actively engaged in monitoring and responding to potential biological threats.

However, the effectiveness of these efforts remains a subject of debate. Verification of compliance with the BWC is challenging, and the potential for non-state actors to acquire and use bioweapons is a persistent concern.

The science of biological warfare is a complex and multifaceted topic with a long history of development and use. While international efforts have sought to prohibit and regulate the use of bioweapons, the challenges posed by modern science and technology underscore the need for continued vigilance and preparedness. The potential consequences of a biological attack are grave, making it imperative that the global community remains committed to preventing the use of biological agents as weapons of mass destruction. Ethical considerations must guide our actions in this field, with a focus on the responsible use of biotechnology for the betterment of humanity rather than its harm.

Understanding Pathogens

Pathogens are microscopic organisms that can cause diseases in humans, animals, and plants. They come in various forms, including bacteria, viruses, fungi, and parasites. Understanding pathogens is crucial for preventing and treating infectious diseases, which have been a significant threat to human health throughout history. In this comprehensive exploration, we will delve into the world of pathogens, examining their types, transmission, the human immune response, and strategies for prevention and treatment.

I. Types of Pathogens

A. Bacteria

Bacteria are single-celled organisms with diverse shapes and characteristics. While many bacteria are harmless or even beneficial to humans, some can cause diseases. Pathogenic bacteria include notorious species like Streptococcus, Escherichia coli (E. coli), and Mycobacterium tuberculosis. These bacteria can infect various parts of the body, leading to conditions ranging from strep throat to tuberculosis.

1.   Streptococcus

Streptococcus bacteria are responsible for a wide range of infections, from minor skin infections to severe illnesses like streptococcal pharyngitis (strep throat) and necrotizing fasciitis (a flesh-eating disease). Understanding different Streptococcus strains and their virulence factors is essential for effective treatment.

2.   Escherichia coli (E. coli)

E. coli is a common inhabitant of the human intestine, but certain strains can cause foodborne illnesses and urinary tract infections (UTIs). E. coli's ability to produce toxins makes it particularly concerning, as it can lead to severe health complications.

3.   Mycobacterium tuberculosis

M. tuberculosis is the bacterium responsible for tuberculosis (TB), a disease that has plagued humanity for centuries. TB remains a significant global health concern, with millions of cases reported annually.

B. Viruses

Viruses are microscopic infectious agents that cannot survive or replicate without a host cell. They come in various shapes and sizes, with the common cold virus, influenza virus, and HIV (human immunodeficiency virus) being well-known examples.

1.   Influenza Virus

Influenza, or the flu, is caused by influenza viruses. These rapidly mutating pathogens pose a continuous challenge for public health due to the need for annual vaccine updates to combat new strains.

2.   Human Immunodeficiency Virus (HIV)

HIV is responsible for acquired immunodeficiency syndrome (AIDS), a condition that weakens the immune system and leaves the body vulnerable to other infections and diseases. Understanding HIV transmission and prevention has been crucial in reducing its global impact.

3.   Coronavirus

Coronaviruses, including SARS-CoV-2, which causes COVID-19, have recently gained global attention. The rapid spread of COVID-19 underscored the importance of understanding virus transmission and developing effective vaccines.

C. Fungi

Fungi are eukaryotic microorganisms that include yeasts, molds, and mushrooms. While most fungi are harmless, some can cause fungal infections, particularly in individuals with weakened immune systems.

1.   Candida

Candida species are commonly found on the skin and mucous membranes, but they can cause infections like oral thrush and vaginal yeast infections when they overgrow.

2.   Aspergillus

Aspergillus species are ubiquitous in the environment and can cause lung infections, particularly in people with underlying lung conditions.

D. Parasites

Parasites are organisms that live in or on another organism (the host) and rely on the host for nutrients. Parasitic infections can affect various parts of the body and can be caused by protozoa, helminths (worms), and arthropods.

1.   Malaria

Malaria, caused by the Plasmodium parasite, is a mosquito-borne disease responsible for millions of deaths worldwide. Understanding the life cycle of the parasite and the behavior of the mosquito vector is essential for malaria control.

2.   Schistosomiasis

Schistosomiasis is caused by parasitic flatworms called schistosomes. These worms can cause chronic and debilitating infections when they penetrate the skin while swimming in contaminated water.

II. Pathogen Transmission

Pathogens have various mechanisms for transmission from one host to another. Understanding these transmission routes is essential for preventing the spread of infectious diseases.

A. Airborne Transmission

Airborne pathogens, such as those causing tuberculosis, influenza, and COVID-19, can be transmitted through respiratory droplets expelled when an infected person coughs, sneezes, or talks.

B. Vector-Borne Transmission

Vector-borne pathogens are transmitted by vectors, such as mosquitoes, ticks, and fleas. These vectors can carry pathogens from one host to another through their bites.

C. Fecal-Oral Transmission

Pathogens like E. coli and hepatitis A can be transmitted through contaminated food, water, or surfaces that have come into contact with fecal matter.

D. Direct Contact Transmission

Some pathogens are transmitted through direct physical contact with an infected person, animal, or surface. Sexually transmitted infections (STIs) like HIV fall into this category.

E. Vertical Transmission

Vertical transmission occurs from mother to child during pregnancy, childbirth, or breastfeeding. It is responsible for the transmission of diseases like HIV and syphilis from mother to child.

F. Indirect Contact Transmission

Indirect contact transmission involves pathogens being transmitted via intermediate objects or surfaces, such as doorknobs or shared utensils.

III. The Human Immune Response

The human immune system is a complex network of cells and molecules that defends the body against pathogens. Understanding how the immune system works is crucial for developing vaccines and treatments.

A. Innate Immunity

Innate immunity is the body's first line of defense against pathogens. It includes physical barriers like the skin, as well as immune cells that can quickly respond to infections.

B. Adaptive Immunity

Adaptive immunity is a more specific and targeted immune response. It involves the production of antibodies and the activation of immune cells that can "remember" and respond more effectively to previously encountered pathogens.

C. Vaccination

Vaccination is a critical tool in the fight against infectious diseases. It works by stimulating the immune system to produce a protective response without causing the disease itself. Understanding the principles of vaccination is essential for controlling epidemics and pandemics.

IV. Prevention and Treatment

Preventing and treating infectious diseases require a multifaceted approach that includes public health measures, antimicrobial medications, and supportive care.

A. Public Health Measures

1.   Hygiene and Sanitation

Basic hygiene practices, such as handwashing with soap and access to clean water, are fundamental in preventing the spread of infectious diseases, particularly in areas with limited resources.

2.   Quarantine and Isolation

Quarantine and isolation measures are crucial for containing outbreaks. Understanding the appropriate use of these measures can help prevent the rapid spread of pathogens.

3.   Vaccination Campaigns

Mass vaccination campaigns are essential for achieving herd immunity and preventing the spread of vaccine-preventable diseases.

B. Antimicrobial Medications

1.   Antibiotics

Antibiotics are used to treat bacterial infections by targeting specific bacterial structures or functions. Understanding antibiotic resistance and the responsible use of antibiotics is vital to combat the growing problem of drug-resistant bacteria.

2.   Antiviral Drugs

Antiviral drugs are used to treat viral infections. They can inhibit viral replication or help manage symptoms. Developing effective antiviral drugs is crucial for combating diseases like HIV and influenza.

C. Supportive Care

Support ive care plays a vital role in managing infectious diseases, particularly those caused by pathogens for which no specific antiviral or antibacterial treatment exists.

1.   Fluid and Nutrient Support

Patients with severe infections often require intravenous fluids and nutritional support to maintain their hydration and energy levels. Understanding the nutritional needs of patients during illness is essential for their recovery.

2.   Symptomatic Treatment

Many infectious diseases come with specific symptoms such as fever, cough, or diarrhea. Providing medications or interventions to alleviate these symptoms can improve the patient's comfort and aid in their recovery.

D. Emerging Therapies

Ongoing research into infectious diseases has led to the development of new therapies and treatment approaches.

1.   Monoclonal Antibodies

Monoclonal antibodies are engineered proteins that can target specific pathogens. They have been used effectively in treating diseases like COVID-19 by neutralizing the virus.

2.   CRISPR Technology

CRISPR technology shows promise in combating infectious diseases by allowing for the precise editing of an organism's DNA, potentially disabling or altering the genes of pathogens.

V. Challenges in Pathogen Understanding

Despite significant progress in understanding and combatting pathogens, several challenges persist.

A. Antimicrobial Resistance

The overuse and misuse of antibiotics have led to the rise of antimicrobial resistance, making it harder to treat bacterial infections. Understanding the mechanisms of resistance and developing alternative treatments is critical.

B. Emerging Infectious Diseases

New infectious diseases continue to emerge, often crossing species barriers. These zoonotic diseases, such as Ebola and COVID-19, highlight the need for a better understanding of the dynamics of pathogen transmission from animals to humans.

C. Vaccine Hesitancy

Vaccine hesitancy, fueled by misinformation and mistrust, poses a significant challenge to vaccination campaigns. Understanding the factors influencing vaccine hesitancy is essential for public health efforts.

D. Global Health Inequality

Access to healthcare, vaccines, and treatments is not equitable worldwide. Bridging the gap in global health inequality is crucial to effectively combatting infectious diseases.

Understanding pathogens is an ongoing and multifaceted endeavor that spans microbiology, immunology, epidemiology, and public health. The ability to identify, track, and respond to infectious diseases is essential for the well-being of individuals and communities around the world.

As we continue to face emerging infectious diseases and the challenge of antimicrobial resistance, research and collaboration among scientists, healthcare professionals, and policymakers remain critical. Equally important is the role of education in raising public awareness about the importance of vaccination, hygiene, and responsible antibiotic use.

The fight against pathogens is a dynamic process, one that requires adaptability, innovation, and a global commitment to ensuring the health and safety of all. By deepening our understanding of pathogens and their impact on human health, we can better prepare for the infectious challenges of the future and work towards a healthier, more resilient world.

Bacteria, Viruses, and Toxins: Unveiling the Microbial World

In the microscopic world, three formidable entities often take center stage: bacteria, viruses, and toxins. These minute agents wield significant influence over life on Earth, from the maintenance of our health to the causes of disease outbreaks. This comprehensive exploration delves into the nature, characteristics, roles, and impacts of these microorganisms, shedding light on the intricate dance between them and the human species.

Bacteria: The Microscopic Powerhouses

What Are Bacteria?

Bacteria are among the most ancient and diverse life forms on Earth. These single-celled organisms are found everywhere, from the deepest oceans to the highest mountains. They come in various shapes, including spheres (cocci), rods (bacilli), and spirals (spirilla). Unlike eukaryotes, bacteria lack a nucleus and other membrane-bound organelles, yet they thrive through astonishing adaptability.

Role of Bacteria

1.   Beneficial Bacteria: Not all bacteria are harmful. In fact, many play vital roles in ecosystems and human life. Soil bacteria facilitate nutrient cycling, while gut bacteria aid in digestion and support the immune system.

2.   Pathogenic Bacteria: Some bacteria can cause diseases in humans and other organisms. Pathogens like Escherichia coli (E. coli) and Streptococcus pneumoniae are responsible for a range of illnesses.

3.   Biotechnology: Bacteria are harnessed in various biotechnological applications, such as the production of antibiotics, insulin, and genetic engineering techniques like CRISPR-Cas9.

The Battle Against Bacterial Infections

The discovery of antibiotics revolutionized medicine, providing effective tools to combat bacterial infections. However, the overuse and misuse of antibiotics have led to antibiotic resistance, a growing global health concern. Innovations in bacteriophage therapy and the development of new antibiotics remain crucial in this ongoing battle.

Viruses: The Masters of Intrusion

What Are Viruses?

Viruses are enigmatic entities that exist in a gray area between life and non-life. They consist of genetic material (DNA or RNA) enclosed in a protein coat called a capsid. Lacking cellular machinery, viruses cannot reproduce on their own and must hijack host cells to replicate.

Viral Diversity

Viruses infect a staggering range of organisms, including bacteria (bacteriophages), plants, animals, and humans. The diversity of viruses is mind-boggling, and they have played significant roles in shaping evolution and ecosystems.

Viral Infections

1.   Common Viral Infections: Many everyday illnesses, from the common cold (rhinovirus) to influenza (influenza virus), are caused by viruses. These infections can range from mild nuisances to life-threatening diseases.

2.   Emerging Viral Threats: The emergence of novel viruses, such as HIV, SARS-CoV-2 (the virus responsible for COVID-19), and Ebola, highlights the ongoing risk posed by viral infections and the need for global preparedness.

Vaccines: A Shield Against Viral Onslaught

Vaccines represent humanity's most potent weapon against viral diseases. They stimulate the immune system to produce antibodies without causing illness, creating immunity and preventing widespread outbreaks.

Toxins: Nature's Hidden Dangers

What Are Toxins?

Toxins are substances produced by living organisms, including bacteria, plants, and animals, that can harm or kill other organisms. They serve various purposes, from defense to predation. Toxins can be categorized as biological, chemical, or environmental.

Types of Toxins

1.   Bacterial Toxins: Bacteria secrete toxins, such as botulinum toxin and tetanus toxin, which can cause severe diseases when introduced into the human body.

2.   Plant Toxins: Many plants contain toxins to deter herbivores. Examples include cyanogenic glycosides in cassava and solanine in potatoes.

3.   Animal Toxins: Venomous animals, such as snakes, spiders, and cone snails, produce toxins that can be lethal to their prey or potential threats.

The Battle Against Toxins

Understanding toxins is crucial for preventing poisoning incidents. Antivenoms, toxin-binding drugs, and detoxification techniques are some of the strategies employed to counteract toxin effects.

Interplay Between Bacteria, Viruses, and Toxins

Microbial Communities

Microbes rarely exist in isolation. In the human body, for instance, a complex ecosystem of bacteria, viruses, and other microorganisms called the microbiome coexists. This intricate balance is essential for maintaining health and preventing infections.

Toxins in Microbial Warfare

Bacteria often employ toxins to compete with other microbes for resources. The battle between bacteria can shape ecosystems and influence the progression of diseases.

Viruses as Biological Weapons

Viruses have been used as tools in biotechnology and, regrettably, as biological weapons. Understanding their biology is crucial for both scientific advancements and global security.

The world of bacteria, viruses, and toxins is a realm of remarkable complexity and adaptability. These microorganisms influence our lives in countless ways, from the beneficial bacteria in our gut to the devastating impact of viral pandemics. To navigate this intricate web of interactions and harness the potential benefits while mitigating the risks, science and society must continue to collaborate and evolve.

In the ongoing battle against infectious diseases and toxins, knowledge remains our most potent weapon. As we delve deeper into the microscopic world, we inch closer to a future where we can harness the power of these entities for the betterment of humanity while safeguarding ourselves against their potential threats.

Weaponization of Biological Agents

The weaponization of biological agents represents a dark and ominous chapter in the history of warfare and global security. It involves the deliberate use of disease-causing microorganisms or toxins as tools of destruction, either to harm humans, animals, or crops. The potential for catastrophic consequences is immense, as biological agents can spread rapidly, remain difficult to trace, and cause widespread illness or death. This essay explores the historical context, methods, motivations, and implications of the weaponization of biological agents, shedding light on the complex ethical, political, and scientific aspects of this perilous endeavor.

I. Historical Context

1.   Early Instances of Biological Warfare

The history of biological warfare dates back centuries. In antiquity, armies would contaminate the water supply of their adversaries with feces or the bodies of plague victims. However, it was during the 20th century that significant developments in the weaponization of biological agents occurred.

2.   World War I and Biological Weapons

During World War I, several nations explored the use of biological agents as weapons, including anthrax and cholera. The use of chemical weapons in this conflict led to the belief that biological warfare might offer a more covert and devastating option.

3.   World War II and Japanese Experiments

Perhaps the most infamous example of biological warfare experimentation occurred during World War II when the Imperial Japanese Army conducted horrific experiments on prisoners of war. Unit 731, led by Dr. Shiro Ishii, conducted experiments with various deadly pathogens, including anthrax and bubonic plague, with devastating consequences.

4.   Cold War and Bioweapons Programs

The Cold War era saw both the United States and the Soviet Union engage in extensive bioweapons research. The U.S. Army's Biological Warfare Laboratories at Fort Detrick,

Maryland, developed a range of biological agents for potential use. This period marked significant advancements in the science and technology of bioweapons.

II. Methods of Weaponization

1.   Types of Biological Agents

Biological agents used as weapons can be categorized into bacteria, viruses, toxins, and fungi. These agents are chosen for their high infectivity, virulence, and potential to cause widespread harm.

2.   Delivery Systems

The effective deployment of biological agents often requires sophisticated delivery systems. These can include aerosol sprays, contaminated food or water supplies, or even infected individuals acting as vectors.

3.   Genetic Engineering

Advancements in genetic engineering have raised concerns about the potential creation of designer pathogens. Scientists can modify existing organisms to make them more lethal, drug-resistant, or immune to existing treatments.

III. Motivations for Weaponization

1.   Military Advantage

One primary motivation for the weaponization of biological agents is the potential for gaining a significant military advantage. Biological weapons can incapacitate an adversary's military and civilian populations, disrupting their ability to wage war.

2.   Covert Warfare

Biological agents offer a level of secrecy and deniability that other weapons may lack. Unlike a missile strike, a bioweapon attack may take days or even weeks to be identified, allowing the aggressor to escape detection.

3.   Terrorist Threat

Non-state actors, such as terrorist organizations, may seek to obtain and use biological agents to instill fear and chaos. The unpredictable nature of biological weapons makes them an attractive choice for those seeking to disrupt society.

IV. International Efforts to Prevent Biological Weaponization

1.   Biological Weapons Convention (BWC)

The BWC, established in 1972, is a multilateral treaty aimed at prohibiting the development, production, and acquisition of biological weapons. It also mandates the destruction of existing stockpiles. However, verification and enforcement have proven challenging.

2.   The Role of International Organizations

Organizations like the World Health Organization (WHO) and the Organization for the Prohibition of Chemical Weapons (OPCW) play vital roles in monitoring and responding to suspected cases of biological weapon use. Their work includes investigating disease outbreaks and conducting inspections of facilities.

3.   Dual-Use Dilemma

One of the challenges in preventing the weaponization of biological agents is the dual-use dilemma. Many scientific advancements that have legitimate medical or research applications can also be misused for bioweapon development.

V. Case Studies

1.   The Aum Shinrikyo Cult

The Aum Shinrikyo cult in Japan attempted to use biological agents, including anthrax and botulinum toxin, in terrorist attacks in the 1990s. Although these attempts were largely unsuccessful, they highlighted the threat posed by non-state actors.

2.   The Amerithrax Attacks

In 2001, the United States experienced a series of anthrax attacks through contaminated letters. The source of these attacks was traced back to a U.S. Army bioweapons researcher, Dr. Bruce Ivins, who committed suicide before being charged.

3.   Allegations of State-Sponsored Bioweapons Programs

There have been allegations of state-sponsored bioweapons programs in countries like North Korea and Syria. These allegations underscore the ongoing challenges of monitoring and verifying compliance with the BWC.

VI. Ethical and Moral Considerations

1.   Humanitarian Concerns

The use of biological weapons raises profound ethical concerns due to the indiscriminate harm they cause. Biological agents do not distinguish between combatants and non-combatants, and their effects can be long-lasting.

2.   The Slippery Slope of Research

The pursuit of knowledge in the life sciences is essential for medical progress, but it can also lead to unintended consequences. Striking a balance between scientific research and security concerns is a persistent ethical challenge.

VII. Future Challenges and Concerns

1.   Advances in Synthetic Biology

Advancements in synthetic biology and gene editing technologies may make it easier for malicious actors to create novel biological weapons. The ability to design custom pathogens raises concerns about the emergence of new bioweapons.

2.   Pandemic Preparedness

The ongoing threat of naturally occurring pandemics, such as the COVID-19 pandemic, underscores the importance of global pandemic preparedness. The skills and infrastructure required to respond to a bioweapon attack are similar to those needed for natural pandemics.

3.   International Cooperation

Preventing the weaponization of biological agents requires international cooperation, information sharing, and diplomacy. Global efforts must strengthen mechanisms for detecting and deterring bioweapon threats.

The weaponization of biological agents represents a chilling convergence of science, security, and ethics. While international treaties and organizations seek to prevent their use, the allure of bioweapons endures. Continued vigilance, regulation, and ethical reflection are essential to navigate the complex terrain of biological warfare in the 21st century. The specter of bioterrorism and the potential for state-sponsored bioweapon programs underscore the need for a united global response to this grave threat to humanity.

The Lethal Potential

Violence, in its many forms, has plagued humanity since the dawn of civilization. It is a destructive force that knows no boundaries, affecting individuals, communities, and nations alike. The lethal potential of violence is a subject of great concern, as it not only claims countless lives but also leaves lasting scars on survivors and society as a whole. This essay explores the multifaceted nature of violence, delving into its root causes, the psychology behind it, its different manifestations, and the ways in which it can be mitigated and prevented. By understanding the lethal potential of violence, we can hope to find ways to curb its devastating impact on our world.

I. The Roots of Violence

A. Biological Factors

Violence, as a behavior, has biological underpinnings. Evolutionary psychology suggests that aggression and violence were once adaptive traits for survival. In our distant past, conflicts over resources and territory often led to violent confrontations. While modern society has evolved, some of these primal instincts still linger within us. Neurobiological studies have identified areas in the brain associated with aggressive behavior, such as the amygdala, and the role of neurotransmitters like serotonin in modulating aggression. However, it's important to note that biology is just one piece of the puzzle, and not all individuals with these biological factors become violent.

B. Social and Environmental Factors

The environment in which a person grows up plays a significant role in shaping their propensity for violence. Poverty, lack of access to education, exposure to violence in the family or community, and peer pressure can all contribute to the development of violent tendencies. The socialization process, which includes the transmission of cultural norms and values, also influences whether a person turns to violence as a means of conflict resolution. The interplay between biological and environmental factors is complex, making it difficult to pinpoint a single cause for violent behavior.

II. The Psychology of Violence

A. Aggression vs. Violence

To understand the lethal potential of violence, it's essential to differentiate between aggression and violence. Aggression refers to any behavior intended to harm another person physically or psychologically, while violence involves the use of force that causes physical harm or damage. While all violent acts are aggressive, not all aggressive acts are violent. Understanding this distinction helps us grasp the continuum of behaviors that can potentially lead to lethal outcomes.

B. The Role of Desensitization

Modern society is saturated with images and narratives of violence, both in real-life news and entertainment media. Exposure to violence, whether real or fictional, can desensitize individuals to its effects. Studies have shown that prolonged exposure to violent media can lead to reduced emotional responsiveness to violence and increased acceptance of aggressive behavior. This desensitization can lower the threshold for engaging in violent acts, contributing to the lethal potential of violence in society.

III. Manifestations of Violence

A. Physical Violence

Physical violence is perhaps the most overt and readily recognizable form of violence. It encompasses a wide range of behaviors, from simple acts of aggression to severe physical harm. Homicide, assault, domestic violence, and acts of terrorism all fall under the umbrella of physical violence. The lethal potential of physical violence is clear, as it can result in death or permanent injury.

B. Psychological Violence

Psychological violence, also known as emotional or mental abuse, is less visible but equally damaging. It involves behaviors aimed at controlling, demeaning, or manipulating another person's thoughts and emotions. Psychological violence can have long-lasting effects on victims, eroding their self-esteem and mental well-being. In extreme cases, it can contribute to the development of conditions like post-traumatic stress disorder (PTSD).

C. Structural Violence

Structural violence refers to the systematic ways in which social, economic, and political structures harm individuals or groups. It is often less overt than physical violence but can be just as lethal. Poverty, discrimination, lack of access to healthcare, and unequal access to education are all examples of structural violence. Such inequities can lead to premature death, illness, and suffering on a large scale.

IV. Preventing and Mitigating Violence

A. Education and Awareness

Education is a powerful tool for preventing violence. Teaching conflict resolution skills, empathy, and communication from an early age can help individuals manage their emotions and resolve conflicts nonviolently. Additionally, raising awareness about the consequences of violence and the available resources for victims can encourage people to seek help and support.

B. Economic and Social Interventions

Addressing the root causes of violence requires targeted economic and social interventions. Programs that alleviate poverty, improve access to quality education, and provide opportunities for skill development can help reduce the likelihood of individuals resorting to violence due to desperation or lack of options. Additionally, addressing systemic inequalities and discrimination can help reduce structural violence.

C. Mental Health Support

Many individuals who engage in violent behavior have underlying mental health issues. Providing accessible and stigma-free mental health support can help identify and address these issues before they escalate into violence. Early intervention and treatment can be crucial in preventing violent acts.

D. Legal and Policy Measures

Effective legal and policy measures can deter violence and hold perpetrators accountable. Stricter gun control laws, restraining orders in cases of domestic violence, and anti-bullying policies in schools are examples of measures aimed at preventing violence. However, it's essential to strike a balance between individual rights and public safety in implementing such measures.

The lethal potential of violence is a complex and multifaceted issue that cannot be fully addressed through a single approach. It requires a comprehensive understanding of the biological, psychological, social, and environmental factors that contribute to violent behavior. By addressing the root causes of violence, raising awareness, and implementing a combination of educational, economic, and legal measures, society can work towards reducing its lethal impact. While violence may always be a part of the human experience, our collective efforts can significantly diminish its destructive potential and create a safer, more compassionate world for future generations.

Biological Agents and Their Effects

Biological agents, often referred to as bioagents or bioweapons, represent a class of weapons that harness the power of living organisms or their byproducts to inflict harm on humans, animals, or plants. The use of biological agents dates back centuries, with various historical accounts documenting instances of warfare involving pathogens, toxins, and even animal vectors. In the modern era, the threat posed by biological agents has garnered significant attention due to advancements in biotechnology and the potential for these agents to cause widespread harm. This essay will delve into the world of biological agents, exploring their various forms, effects, and the implications for security and public health.

I. Classification of Biological Agents

Biological agents can be categorized into several distinct classes based on their origin, purpose, and mode of action. The main categories include:

1.   Pathogens: Pathogenic microorganisms, such as bacteria, viruses, fungi, and protozoa, are the most widely recognized biological agents. These organisms can cause diseases in humans, animals, or plants. Examples include anthrax (caused by Bacillus anthracis), smallpox (variola virus), and botulism (Clostridium botulinum).
2.   Toxins: Toxins are poisonous substances produced by certain organisms. They can be derived from bacteria (e.g., botulinum toxin), plants (e.g., ricin), or animals (e.g., snake venom). Toxins are potent and can cause severe illness or death.
3.   Bioregulators: Bioregulators are chemicals that disrupt normal biological processes. For instance, organophosphates like sarin interfere with neurotransmission, leading to paralysis and death. These agents can be synthetic or naturally occurring.
4.   Vectors: Some biological agents employ living organisms, such as insects, to transmit diseases. Malaria, for example, is transmitted by female Anopheles mosquitoes carrying the Plasmodium parasite.

II. Effects of Biological Agents

The effects of biological agents on living organisms can be devastating. The impact varies depending on the type of agent, its virulence, and the host's susceptibility. Here are some common effects:

1.   Disease Outbreaks: Pathogens are often used as biological agents to induce disease outbreaks. When released intentionally, they can cause epidemics or pandemics, overwhelming healthcare systems and leading to high mortality rates.

2.   Toxicity: Toxins, whether natural or synthetic, can cause severe poisoning in humans and animals. Symptoms may include nausea, vomiting, paralysis, convulsions, and death in extreme cases.

3.   Long-Term Health Effects: Exposure to certain biological agents can result in long-term health consequences. For example, survivors of anthrax attacks may experience chronic health issues, including lung damage and fatigue.

4.   Environmental Damage: Biological agents can also target plants and animals. Crop pathogens, for instance, can destroy agricultural crops, leading to food shortages, economic losses, and ecological imbalances.

5.   Psychological Impact: Beyond physical harm, the fear and uncertainty associated with biological agents can have a profound psychological impact on affected populations. This psychological trauma can persist long after the initial exposure.

III. Historical Use of Biological Agents

Throughout history, various civilizations and military forces have employed biological agents as weapons. Here are some notable examples:

1.   Siege of Caffa (1346): During the siege of Caffa (now Feodosiya, Ukraine), the Mongol army catapulted plague-infected corpses over the city walls, leading to an outbreak of the Black Death inside the city.

2.   World War I: Both the Allied and Central Powers researched the use of biological agents during World War I. The Germans, in particular, are known to have used anthrax and glanders as potential weapons.

3.   World War II: The Japanese Imperial Army conducted extensive biological warfare research during World War II, including experiments on prisoners of war. They used agents like plague and anthrax in China.

4.   Cold War Era: The United States and the Soviet Union developed extensive biological weapons programs during the Cold War. The Biological Weapons Convention (BWC) of 1972 aimed to curb these programs, leading to the destruction of stockpiles and the cessation of offensive biological weapons development.

IV. Contemporary Threats

While the use of biological agents as weapons has decreased since the signing of the BWC, the threat persists due to several factors:

1.   Biotechnology Advancements: Advances in biotechnology have made it easier to manipulate and engineer microorganisms. This increases the potential for the creation of novel, more potent biological agents.

2.   Dual-Use Research: Some scientific research, while intended for beneficial purposes, can have dual-use potential, meaning it could also be used for harmful purposes. This dual-use nature complicates efforts to regulate and secure biological research.

3.   Bioterrorism: Terrorist groups or individuals with access to biological agents and knowledge could use them to carry out attacks. These attacks could target civilian populations or critical infrastructure.

4.   Accidental Releases: Laboratories and facilities conducting research on biological agents face the risk of accidental releases, which could lead to unintended outbreaks.

5.   Emerging Diseases: Natural pathogens, such as novel viruses, can also pose significant threats. The COVID-19 pandemic serves as a stark reminder of the global impact of emerging diseases.

V. Security and Preparedness

Given the ongoing threat posed by biological agents, governments and international organizations have taken measures to enhance security and preparedness:

1.   Biological Weapons Convention (BWC): The BWC is a crucial international treaty that prohibits the development, production, and stockpiling of biological weapons. It also promotes transparency and cooperation among member states.

2.   Biosecurity Measures: Laboratories working with dangerous pathogens are expected to adhere to strict biosecurity protocols to prevent accidental releases and unauthorized access.

3.   Surveillance and Early Warning: Global surveillance networks monitor disease outbreaks and unusual patterns of illness to detect potential biological agent use promptly.

4.   Response Planning: Governments and organizations have developed response plans to manage biological agent incidents, including the distribution of medical countermeasures and public health measures.

5.   Research Oversight: Oversight mechanisms are in place to review and regulate potentially dual-use research to prevent misuse.

VI. Ethical and Legal Considerations

The use of biological agents as weapons raises profound ethical and legal questions:

1.   Moral Responsibility: The deliberate use of biological agents to harm civilians or combatants is widely considered morally reprehensible, and perpetrators may face condemnation and prosecution.

2.   Accountability: Identifying the source of a biological attack can be challenging. Establishing accountability is critical for legal and diplomatic responses.

3.   Dual-Use Dilemma: Balancing scientific research for beneficial purposes with the potential for misuse presents an ongoing ethical challenge. Striking this balance requires international cooperation and guidelines.

4.   Preparedness vs. Deterrence: Nations must balance preparedness against the risk of provoking conflict. Overemphasis on preparedness can lead to mistrust and escalation, while underemphasizing it risks leaving populations vulnerable.

Biological agents, whether naturally occurring or engineered, represent a potent and complex threat to human and environmental health. While the use of biological weapons has decreased since the signing of the Biological Weapons Convention, the potential for misuse remains a pressing concern. Advancements in biotechnology, the dual-use nature of research, and the threat of bioterrorism all require ongoing vigilance and international cooperation.

Addressing the challenge of biological agents requires a multifaceted approach, encompassing robust surveillance, response planning, research oversight, and a commitment to ethical and legal principles. It is essential to strike a balance between protecting public health and ensuring security without stifling legitimate scientific progress.

One of the key takeaways from the history of biological agents is the need for international cooperation. Given the global nature of biological threats, no single nation can effectively address the risks in isolation. International agreements and organizations play a critical role in fostering collaboration and setting standards.

As we move forward, several areas require continued attention and action:

1.   Enhanced Surveillance and Detection: Advances in data analytics, genomics, and epidemiology can significantly improve our ability to detect and respond to biological threats. Governments and organizations should invest in robust surveillance systems to monitor and analyze emerging diseases and unusual patterns of illness.

2.   Public Health Infrastructure: Strengthening public health infrastructure is vital for effective response to biological threats. This includes building capacity for rapid diagnosis, contact tracing, and vaccination campaigns in the event of an outbreak.

3.   Research Ethics and Oversight: The scientific community must continue to develop and adhere to ethical guidelines for research involving potentially dual-use technologies. Oversight mechanisms should be enhanced to prevent accidental releases and ensure responsible conduct.

4.   Global Cooperation: International cooperation remains essential for addressing biological threats. This includes sharing information, resources, and expertise to respond to outbreaks and prevent bioterrorism.

5.   Education and Awareness: Public awareness and education about biological threats are crucial. An informed public is better equipped to recognize unusual health patterns and support measures to prevent the misuse of biological agents.

6.   Policy and Diplomacy: Governments should continue to engage in diplomacy to strengthen international agreements, such as the Biological Weapons Convention, and to hold violators accountable. Policymakers must also strike a balance between preparedness and deterrence.

7.   Innovation and Research: Research into new medical countermeasures, diagnostics, and vaccines for potential biological agents is ongoing. Investment in innovation is critical to stay ahead of evolving threats.

8.   Crisis Communication: Effective communication during biological events is vital to prevent panic and ensure public trust. Governments and organizations should have well-prepared communication strategies in place.

In conclusion, biological agents represent a complex and ever-evolving challenge to global security and public health. While history provides us with stark reminders of the devastating potential of these agents, it also demonstrates our capacity to respond and adapt. Through international cooperation, research ethics, preparedness measures, and a commitment to the well-being of all, we can continue to mitigate the risks posed by biological agents and work towards a safer, more secure world. It is a challenge that demands ongoing vigilance, innovation, and a shared sense of responsibility for the well-being of humanity.

Mechanisms of Infection and Transmission

Infectious diseases have been a constant companion of humanity throughout history. Understanding the mechanisms of infection and transmission is crucial for public health, as it allows us to develop strategies to control and prevent the spread of these diseases. This article explores the fundamental mechanisms behind infection and transmission, shedding light on how pathogens invade the body and how they are passed from person to person.

I. Pathogens: The Microscopic Invaders

Pathogens are microorganisms capable of causing disease in their hosts. They come in various forms, including bacteria, viruses, fungi, and parasites. Each type of pathogen has unique mechanisms of infection and transmission, but they share common strategies for survival and replication.

A. Bacteria

1.   Adhesion and Colonization
•   Bacterial pathogens often have specific adhesion molecules that allow them to attach to host cells.
•   Once attached, they colonize and multiply, often forming biofilms for protection.
2.   Invasion
•   Some bacteria have evolved mechanisms to invade host cells, either through direct penetration or by hijacking host cell processes.
3.   Toxins
•   Many bacterial infections result from the production and release of toxins, which damage host tissues and contribute to disease symptoms.

B. Viruses

1.   Attachment and Entry
•   Viruses use specialized proteins or receptors to attach to host cell surfaces.
•   They then enter the host cell, often by fusion with the cell membrane or endocytosis.
2.   Replication
•   Viruses lack cellular machinery, so they rely on host cell machinery to replicate.
•   This often leads to host cell damage and cell death.
3.   Evasion of Immune Response
•   Viruses can evade the immune system by mutating rapidly or inhibiting host immune responses.

C. Fungi

1.   Adhesion and Penetration
•   Fungal pathogens may adhere to host tissues and penetrate them using specialized structures like hyphae.
2.   Tissue Invasion
•   Some fungi can invade deeper tissues, causing severe infections.
3.   Immune Evasion
•   Fungi can evade host immune responses by altering their surface proteins or secreting toxins.

D. Parasites

1.   Entry and Migration
•   Parasites often enter the host through vectors like mosquitoes or contaminated food and water.
•   They may migrate through tissues and organs, causing damage along the way.
2.   Reproduction
•   Parasites reproduce within the host, sometimes leading to the formation of cysts or larvae.

II. Transmission: From Host to Host

Once pathogens have successfully infected a host, they often need to find a new host to continue their life cycle. The mechanisms of transmission vary widely between different pathogens.

A. Direct Transmission

1.   Person-to-Person
•   Many infectious diseases spread through close contact between infected and uninfected individuals.
•   Examples include respiratory infections like the flu and COVID-19.
2.   Sexual Transmission
•   Sexually transmitted infections (STIs) are spread through sexual contact.
•   Proper use of barrier methods like condoms can reduce transmission risk.
3.   Vertical Transmission
•   Some pathogens can be passed from mother to child during childbirth or through breastfeeding.
•   Examples include HIV and certain bacterial infections.

B. Indirect Transmission

1.   Airborne Transmission
•   Pathogens can become airborne in respiratory droplets, remaining suspended in the air.
•   Examples include tuberculosis and measles.
2.   Waterborne Transmission
•   Contaminated water sources can harbor pathogens, leading to waterborne diseases like cholera and giardiasis.
3.   Vector-Borne Transmission
•   Vectors such as mosquitoes and ticks can carry and transmit pathogens.
•   Examples include malaria and Lyme disease.
4.   Fomite Transmission
•   Pathogens can survive on surfaces and objects, leading to transmission when people touch contaminated surfaces.
•   Regular hand hygiene is essential to prevent fomite transmission.

III. Host Factors in Infection and Transmission

The susceptibility of individuals to infection and their ability to transmit pathogens are influenced by various host factors.

A. Immune Response

•   A robust immune system can prevent infection or limit its severity.
•   Immunization can enhance immunity against specific pathogens.

B. Age and Health

•   Infants, the elderly, and individuals with underlying health conditions are often more susceptible to infections.
•   Healthy lifestyles can bolster resistance to infections.

C. Genetic Factors

•   Genetic variations can impact susceptibility to certain infections.
•   Some individuals may have genetic immunity or increased vulnerability.

IV. Control and Prevention

Understanding the mechanisms of infection and transmission is crucial for developing effective strategies to control and prevent the spread of infectious diseases.

A. Vaccination

• Vaccines stimulate the immune system to produce protective antibodies against specific pathogens.

B. Hygiene and Sanitation

• Proper hygiene practices, such as handwashing and sanitation, can reduce the risk of transmission.

C. Antimicrobial Therapies

• Antibiotics, antivirals, and antifungal drugs are essential for treating infections.

D. Vector Control

• Controlling vectors, such as mosquito nets and insecticides, is vital for preventing vector-borne diseases.

E. Education and Public Health Measures

• Public health campaigns can raise awareness and promote behaviors that reduce transmission.

Mechanisms of infection and transmission are complex and diverse, reflecting the incredible adaptability of pathogens and their interaction with host organisms. Understanding these mechanisms is essential for the development of effective prevention and treatment strategies, ultimately reducing the burden of infectious diseases on global health. As our knowledge of pathogens and their interactions with hosts continues to grow, so too will our ability to combat these microscopic invaders.

Historical Perspectives

Biological warfare, the use of infectious agents to harm or incapacitate an enemy, is a dark chapter in human history. Throughout the ages, societies have sought to exploit the inherent vulnerability of populations to diseases, turning them into weapons of mass destruction. This essay delves into the historical perspectives of biological warfare, focusing on the role of epidemic and pandemic outbreaks in shaping the strategies, ethics, and consequences of this perilous form of warfare.

I. Antiquity and Early Uses of Biological Warfare

The origins of biological warfare can be traced back to ancient times when rudimentary knowledge of contagious diseases was used to gain a strategic advantage. In ancient Greece, during the Peloponnesian War (431-404 BCE), Thucydides recorded a plague outbreak in Athens, which had a profound impact on the course of the conflict. It's been suggested that the city's enemies may have intentionally introduced the disease, serving as a grim precursor to future biological warfare tactics.

Similarly, in 1347, as the Black Death swept through Europe, there were suspicions that Mongol armies besieging Caffa (modern-day Feodosiya, Ukraine) used the corpses of plague victims as biological weapons, catapulting them into the city to spread the disease among its inhabitants.

II. The Age of Colonialism and Biological Warfare

During the Age of Colonialism, European powers ventured into new territories, bringing diseases with them that decimated indigenous populations. While many of these introductions were unintentional, there were instances where colonial powers deliberately used biological warfare to subdue native populations.

One notable example is the use of smallpox-infected blankets by British forces during the Pontiac's Rebellion (1763) in North America. This early act of biological warfare aimed to reduce the number of indigenous warriors opposing British expansion.

III. World War I: The Geneva Protocol and the First Modern Bioethical Dilemma

World War I witnessed the first modern attempt to regulate biological warfare. In 1925, the Geneva Protocol banned the use of chemical and biological weapons in warfare. However, the protocol did not prohibit their development or stockpiling, leading to continued research in secret laboratories.

The Geneva Protocol marked the beginning of an ethical debate surrounding biological warfare. While it sought to limit its use, the ambiguity of the protocol's language left room for interpretation, and some nations continued their covert research into biological weapons.

IV. World War II: The Japanese Unit 731 and the Biological Atrocities

One of the most notorious episodes of biological warfare occurred during World War II, when the Japanese Imperial Army's Unit 731 conducted horrific experiments on human subjects in China and other occupied territories. These experiments aimed to develop biological weapons, including plague, anthrax, and cholera, for use against enemy forces.

The scale and brutality of Unit 731's experiments were unprecedented, and they raised profound ethical questions about the limits of scientific research during wartime. The data collected from these experiments remained classified for decades, highlighting the secrecy surrounding biological warfare research.

V. The Cold War Era: Biological Warfare Escalates

The Cold War era witnessed a significant escalation in the development and deployment of biological weapons. Both the United States and the Soviet Union engaged in extensive research and stockpiling of such weapons. The fear of a biological arms race led to the 1972 Biological Weapons Convention (BWC), which sought to prohibit the development, production, and possession of biological weapons.

However, the effectiveness of the BWC was compromised by difficulties in verification and a lack of enforcement mechanisms. Despite the treaty, both superpowers continued their covert research and maintained vast stockpiles of biological agents.

VI. The Biological Weapons Convention: A Fragile Treaty

The Biological Weapons Convention has faced numerous challenges and ambiguities. One of the key issues is the dual-use nature of biological research. While many scientific advancements can benefit humanity, they can also be misused for military purposes.

The rise of biotechnology and genetic engineering in the late 20th century further complicated matters. The potential for engineered pathogens with enhanced virulence or drug resistance raised concerns about the emergence of "designer" biological weapons.

VII. The Anthrax Attacks of 2001: A Wake-Up Call

The anthrax attacks in the United States in 2001 marked a significant turning point in the modern history of biological warfare. Letters containing anthrax spores were sent to media outlets and government offices, resulting in several deaths and widespread panic. These attacks exposed vulnerabilities in the country's biodefense capabilities and raised questions about the accessibility of biological weapons.

The investigation into the attacks revealed that the anthrax used was of domestic origin, originating from a U.S. government laboratory. This incident underscored the need for improved security measures and international cooperation to prevent the illicit acquisition of biological agents.

VIII. Emerging Threats in the 21st Century

The 21st century has brought new challenges in the realm of biological warfare. Advances in biotechnology have made it easier to manipulate genes and create synthetic pathogens. The potential for bioterrorism has increased, raising concerns about the deliberate release of genetically engineered, highly contagious, and drug-resistant pathogens.

Additionally, the COVID-19 pandemic, which emerged in late 2019, highlighted the devastating impact of natural pandemics on global health, economies, and security. The pandemic underscored the need for international cooperation in responding to health crises and raised questions about the intersection of public health and national security.

IX. Ethical Dilemmas and Biosecurity

The use of biological warfare poses profound ethical dilemmas. The deliberate spread of deadly diseases raises questions about the morality of targeting civilian populations and the potential for unintended consequences. It challenges the principles of proportionality and discrimination in warfare.

Biosecurity, the protection of biological agents and research from theft or misuse, has become a critical concern. Laboratories working on dangerous pathogens must balance the need for scientific advancement with the imperative to prevent accidental releases or theft of dangerous materials.

X. The Way Forward: Strengthening the Biological Weapons Convention

In recent years, there have been efforts to strengthen the Biological Weapons Convention. These include proposals for more robust verification mechanisms, increased transparency in biodefense programs, and a renewed commitment to preventing the development and use of biological weapons.

International cooperation in monitoring and responding to disease outbreaks has also gained importance. Initiatives like the Global Health Security Agenda aim to enhance preparedness and response to biological threats while promoting information sharing and collaboration among nations.

Historical perspectives on biological warfare demonstrate the enduring fascination with using diseases as weapons and the complex ethical, political, and security challenges that arise from such practices. While the horrors of past episodes like Unit 731 and the anthrax attacks serve as cautionary tales, the continued advancement of biotechnology presents new threats and uncertainties.

Efforts to strengthen the Biological Weapons Convention and enhance global biosecurity measures are essential steps toward preventing the use of biological weapons in the future. The lessons of history remind us of the catastrophic consequences of biological warfare and the urgent need for vigilance, cooperation, and ethical scrutiny in the realm of biotechnology and biodefense.

Ancient and Medieval Biological Warfare

Biological warfare, the use of infectious agents or toxins as weapons, is a concept that has been part of human history for millennia. While often associated with modern warfare and the development of deadly pathogens in labs, the use of biological agents as weapons has a long and complex history that stretches back to ancient and medieval times. This essay explores the historical context, methods, and consequences of ancient and medieval biological warfare, shedding light on how humanity's early encounters with biological weapons laid the foundation for contemporary discussions on this morally and ethically fraught topic.

I. The Historical Context of Biological Warfare

To understand ancient and medieval biological warfare, it's essential to grasp the historical context in which these practices emerged. The use of infectious agents and toxins as weapons can be traced back to various civilizations, including the Greeks, Romans, and Chinese, who faced threats from rival nations and sought innovative ways to gain military advantages.

A. Ancient Greece and the Use of Disease

In ancient Greece, the city-state of Athens employed a form of biological warfare during the Peloponnesian War (431-404 BCE). Thucydides, an ancient historian, documented how the Athenians forced a devastating plague upon the city of Sparta by contaminating its water sources. While the exact nature of the disease remains a subject of debate among historians, this incident serves as one of the earliest recorded instances of biological warfare.

B. Roman Ingenuity and Deception

The Romans were known for their engineering prowess and cunning tactics, and this extended to warfare. During sieges, they would catapult pots filled with diseased animals or corpses into enemy-held cities, hoping to spread infection. In one famous example, during the siege of Hatra (in modern-day Iraq), the Romans are believed to have catapulted beehives into the city, unleashing a swarm of angry bees as a form of biological attack.

C. Chinese Use of Arsenic and Toxic Smoke

Ancient China also contributed to the early history of biological warfare. The use of arsenic-laced smoke as a weapon dates back to the 4th century BCE. Chinese military strategists and alchemists devised various methods for producing toxic fumes, which they used during sieges to incapacitate or kill enemy forces.

II. Medieval Times: Plague as a Biological Weapon

The medieval period saw the devastating impact of biological warfare in the form of the bubonic plague. The Black Death, as it's commonly known, swept through Europe during the 14th century, killing an estimated 25 million people. While the Black Death is often viewed as a natural pandemic, there is evidence to suggest that it may have been used as a weapon in some instances.

A. The Tartar Siege of Kaffa

One notable case is the siege of Kaffa (now Feodosiya, Ukraine) in 1347-1348. The Tartar army, besieging the city, is said to have catapulted plague-infested corpses over the walls. This gruesome act is believed to have contributed to the outbreak of the Black Death in the city, which then spread to Europe through trade routes.

B. Accidental or Intentional?

Debates persist regarding whether the Tartars intentionally used the plague as a biological weapon or if it was an unintended consequence of the siege. Nevertheless, the siege of Kaffa serves as a compelling historical example of how pathogens can be exploited in warfare.

III. The Consequences of Biological Warfare

The use of biological warfare in ancient and medieval times had profound consequences, both immediate and long-term.

A. Immediate Impact on Military Strategy

The use of biological agents and toxins in warfare altered military strategies. Rulers and generals recognized the potential of these weapons to demoralize, weaken, or even wipe out enemy forces and populations. This led to the development of various techniques and technologies for delivering these agents, including the aforementioned catapults and poisoned smoke.

B. Long-term Societal and Cultural Effects

The fear of biological warfare left a lasting imprint on societies. It contributed to the development of concepts like quarantine and isolation to control disease outbreaks. These practices were initially implemented to protect populations from the unintended consequences of biological warfare, but they evolved into critical public health measures.

C. Ethical and Moral Dilemmas

The use of biological warfare in ancient and medieval times also raised ethical and moral questions. Even in periods of brutal warfare, the deliberate use of diseases or toxins to harm civilians, including women and children, was seen by some as crossing a moral boundary. These ethical dilemmas continue to shape discussions surrounding contemporary biological warfare.

IV. The Legacy of Ancient and Medieval Biological Warfare

The legacy of ancient and medieval biological warfare is still visible in the modern world. While the methods and agents used have evolved, the fundamental principles remain the same. Today, biological warfare is a pressing concern due to advances in science and technology. The lessons from history highlight the importance of addressing this issue ethically and strategically.

A. Modern Biological Warfare

In the 20th and 21st centuries, nations have developed sophisticated biological weapons programs. The most infamous example is the Soviet Union's Biopreparat program, which produced a range of deadly pathogens, including anthrax and smallpox. These programs underscore the potential for catastrophic harm that biological weapons pose.

B. International Efforts to Ban Biological Weapons

Recognizing the grave threat of biological warfare, the international community has taken steps to prevent their use. The Biological Weapons Convention (BWC) of 1972 prohibits the development, production, and acquisition of biological weapons. However, verifying compliance with the treaty remains challenging due to the dual-use nature of many biotechnologies.

C. Ethical Considerations

The historical use of biological warfare raises significant ethical considerations for the modern era. Debates persist regarding the moral boundaries of research into deadly pathogens and the potential dual-use nature of scientific advancements. Striking a balance between scientific progress and global security is a complex challenge.

Ancient and medieval history is replete with instances of biological warfare, where infectious agents and toxins were harnessed as weapons of destruction. These early encounters with biological weapons had profound and lasting effects on military strategy, societal practices, and ethical considerations. As we navigate the complexities of modern biological warfare, it is essential to learn from history and strive for responsible and ethical use of biotechnologies to safeguard global security and human well-being.

Early Instances of Bioweapons

Biological warfare, the use of biological agents to harm or kill an adversary, has a history dating back thousands of years. From ancient times to the modern era, various civilizations have employed bioweapons for strategic advantage. This essay explores the early instances of bioweapons, delving into their origins, tactics, and ethical implications.

1. Antiquity: Early Biological Warfare

1.1. The Siege of Kirrha (590 BC)

One of the earliest recorded instances of bioweapons dates back to ancient Greece. In 590 BC, during the siege of Kirrha, the inhabitants poisoned the water supply with hellebore roots. Hellebore, a toxic plant, caused severe gastrointestinal distress among the besieging forces, ultimately leading to their surrender.

1.2. The Plague of Caffa (1346-1347)

In the 14th century, during the siege of Caffa (now Feodosiya, Ukraine) by Mongol forces, the defenders reportedly catapulted plague-infected corpses over the city walls. This act is considered one of the earliest instances of biological warfare in the form of "biological bombardment." It is believed to have contributed to the spread of the Black Death across Europe.

2. The Age of Exploration: Biological Exchanges

2.1. Smallpox Blankets (18th Century)

During the colonization of the Americas, European settlers and military commanders sought to weaken Native American populations by gifting them blankets contaminated with smallpox. While not a deliberate bioweapon in the modern sense, this practice led to devastating epidemics among indigenous communities, illustrating the unintentional consequences of early biological exchanges.

3. Nineteenth Century: Scientific Advancements

3.1. The Use of Anthrax by Louis Pasteur (1877)

In the late 19th century, the French scientist Louis Pasteur conducted experiments with anthrax, a deadly bacterial disease. His work paved the way for understanding how biological agents could be harnessed for warfare. While Pasteur's intentions were primarily focused on vaccines and prevention, his research had dual-use potential.

4. World War I: The Birth of Modern Bioweapons

4.1. The German Sabotage Program (1915-1918)

During World War I, Germany established a secret program known as the "Sabotage Bureau." This program aimed to disrupt Allied production and demoralize civilian populations through the use of biological agents like anthrax and glanders. Fortunately, these efforts did not result in significant casualties.

5. The Interwar Period: International Agreements

5.1. The Geneva Protocol (1925)

In the aftermath of World War I, the Geneva Protocol was established, prohibiting the use of chemical and biological weapons in warfare. While it did not prevent research and development, it marked a significant step in acknowledging the ethical and humanitarian concerns surrounding bioweapons.

6. World War II: Japan's Biological Warfare Unit 731

6.1. Unit 731 (1937-1945)

Perhaps one of the most notorious instances of bioweapons in the 20th century was Japan's Unit 731. This covert unit conducted gruesome experiments on humans, including the dissemination of deadly pathogens like plague and anthrax in Chinese cities. These actions resulted in the deaths of thousands.

7. The Cold War Era: Bioweapons Programs

7.1. The United States and the Soviet Union

During the Cold War, both the United States and the Soviet Union conducted extensive research into bioweapons. The U.S. program, known as "Project BioShield," aimed to develop countermeasures against potential bioweapon threats. The Soviet Union, on the other hand, had an active bioweapons program, with stockpiles of deadly agents.

8. Contemporary Concerns and Ethical Dilemmas

8.1. The Biological Weapons Convention (BWC) (1972)

The Biological Weapons Convention, which came into force in 1975, reaffirmed the prohibition of bioweapons and mandated the destruction of existing stockpiles. However, compliance and verification have posed significant challenges, and concerns about bioweapon proliferation persist to this day.

8.2. Dual-Use Research

In the 21st century, advances in biotechnology have raised concerns about dual-use research—legitimate scientific research that can have dual applications, both beneficial and harmful. Striking a balance between scientific progress and biosecurity remains an ongoing ethical dilemma.

Early instances of bioweapons reveal the dark side of human ingenuity, where knowledge of biology and disease was sometimes harnessed for destructive purposes. While there have been efforts to control and prohibit bioweapons, the potential for misuse remains a pressing concern in our modern world. Ethical considerations, international agreements, and robust oversight are essential in preventing the resurgence of bioweapons and ensuring a safer future for humanity.

The Use of Plague as a Weapon

Throughout human history, infectious diseases have been used as weapons of war, terror, and subterfuge. One of the most notorious diseases in this regard is the plague, specifically the bubonic plague, caused by the bacterium Yersinia pestis. This disease has a long and dark history, with instances of it being harnessed intentionally for warfare and bioterrorism. This essay explores the historical and contemporary use of the plague as a weapon, the implications it carries, and the efforts to prevent such sinister applications.

I. Historical Use of Plague as a Weapon

1.1. The Siege of Caffa (1347)

One of the earliest documented instances of plague being used as a weapon occurred during the Siege of Caffa, a city on the Crimean Peninsula, in 1347. The Mongol army, besieging the city, suffered from a severe outbreak of the bubonic plague. In an act of desperation, they catapulted the corpses of their plague-infected soldiers over the city walls. This tactic, intended to spread the disease among the besieged population, may have contributed to the rapid transmission of the plague throughout Europe.

1.2. Japanese Biological Warfare Unit 731 (1930s-1940s)

During World War II, the Imperial Japanese Army operated a secretive and horrific biological warfare program known as Unit 731. This unit conducted experiments with various deadly pathogens, including Yersinia pestis. They sought to weaponize the bubonic plague by infecting prisoners and observing the effects of the disease. While their attempts at weaponization were not widely successful, it highlights the potential for state-sponsored bioterrorism.

1.3. Soviet Bioweapons Program (20th Century)

The Soviet Union also had a bioweapons program, which included research on the use of Yersinia pestis as a biological weapon. This program was highly secretive, but it is known that Soviet scientists developed strains of the plague bacterium that were antibiotic-resistant, making them even more deadly. The collapse of the Soviet Union raised concerns about the potential proliferation of such bioweapons.

II. Contemporary Concerns

2.1. Terrorism and Non-State Actors

In the modern era, the threat of plague being used as a weapon has not diminished. Non-state actors, including terrorist organizations, have expressed interest in bioterrorism. The ease of accessing information about biological agents online, coupled with advances in biotechnology, makes it increasingly feasible for individuals or small groups to attempt bioterrorist acts involving plague.

2.2. Laboratory Accidents and Misuse

Laboratories around the world study dangerous pathogens, including Yersinia pestis, for scientific research, vaccine development, and diagnostics. However, there is a constant risk of accidents or misuse in these facilities. A laboratory-acquired infection or an intentional breach could lead to the unintentional release of the plague bacterium into the population.

2.3. Dual-Use Research

The concept of dual-use research refers to scientific experiments or advancements that have both beneficial and harmful potential. In the field of microbiology, research into the genetics and pathogenicity of Yersinia pestis, while intended for understanding and developing treatments, could also be misappropriated for nefarious purposes.

III. Implications and Consequences

3.1. Human Suffering

The use of plague as a weapon carries immense humanitarian consequences. Plague is a highly lethal disease, with a mortality rate approaching 90% if left untreated. Those infected often experience excruciating symptoms, including high fever, swollen lymph nodes (buboes), and septicemia. The deliberate release of such a disease would result in widespread suffering and death.

3.2. Social Disruption

A plague outbreak, whether natural or intentional, can cause profound social disruption. Quarantines, travel restrictions, and panic can lead to economic collapse, strained healthcare systems, and social unrest. The psychological impact of such an event would extend far beyond the physical toll, eroding trust in institutions and sowing fear.

3.3. Global Security

The use of plague as a weapon has significant implications for global security. The proliferation of bioterrorism could lead to a breakdown of international relations and cooperation. Nations may respond aggressively to perceived threats, potentially escalating conflicts.

IV. Prevention and Mitigation

4.1. International Agreements

To counter the threat of bioterrorism, international agreements and treaties have been established. The Biological Weapons Convention (BWC), in force since 1975, bans the development, production, and acquisition of biological weapons. However, enforcing compliance with such agreements remains challenging.

4.2. Biosafety and Biosecurity Measures

Laboratories working with dangerous pathogens must adhere to strict biosafety and biosecurity protocols. These measures include secure storage, controlled access, and rigorous training to prevent accidental releases or unauthorized access to deadly pathogens.

4.3. Surveillance and Early Detection

Early detection is crucial in preventing the intentional release of plague. Surveillance systems, both at a national and international level, are designed to monitor disease outbreaks and identify potential bioterrorist threats.

4.4. Vaccination and Treatment

Efforts to develop effective vaccines and treatments for plague continue. Widespread vaccination could provide a level of immunity in the population, reducing the impact of a deliberate outbreak.

The use of plague as a weapon, whether in historical conflicts or in the contemporary era, remains a troubling and dangerous prospect. The potential for widespread suffering, social disruption, and global instability underscores the urgency of prevention and preparedness efforts. While international agreements and biosafety measures provide some safeguards, vigilance and cooperation among nations are essential to mitigate this grave threat to humanity. The lessons from history should serve as a stark reminder of the destructive power of infectious diseases when harnessed for sinister purposes.

20th Century Biowarfare Programs

The 20th century was a period marked by tremendous advancements in science and technology, but it was also a time when nations engaged in covert and often morally questionable endeavors, including biowarfare programs. Biowarfare, the use of biological agents to harm or kill people, has a long and dark history, with the 20th century witnessing some of its most significant developments. In this exploration, we will delve into the key biowarfare programs of the 20th century, the motivations behind them, the ethical dilemmas they raised, and the global response to this threat.

Section 1: Early 20th Century Precursors

The early 20th century saw the seeds of biowarfare programs being sown, primarily in response to developments in bacteriology and virology. Nations like Germany and the United States began researching the potential military applications of disease-causing agents. The most notable figure in this era was Fritz Haber, a German chemist, who explored the use of chlorine gas during World War I, laying the groundwork for future chemical and biological warfare.

Section 2: World War II and the Japanese Unit 731

The horrors of World War II saw the emergence of more extensive and sinister biowarfare programs. Japan's Unit 731, led by General Shiro Ishii, conducted inhumane experiments on thousands of Chinese, Korean, and Allied prisoners. This research aimed to develop bioweapons like bubonic plague and anthrax. The secrecy and brutality of Unit 731 remain a stain on the annals of history.

Section 3: The Cold War Era

The post-World War II period marked the height of biowarfare research, with the United States and the Soviet Union at the forefront. Both nations believed that biological weapons could be a cost-effective means of mass destruction. The U.S. initiated programs like Operation Paperclip, while the Soviets conducted extensive research on bioweapons like smallpox.

Section 4: International Conventions and the End of Offensive Programs

The atrocities of World War II prompted international efforts to regulate and curtail biowarfare. The Geneva Protocol of 1925 banned the use of biological and chemical weapons in warfare, but enforcement remained weak. The Biological Weapons

Convention of 1972 aimed to strengthen these prohibitions, leading to the eventual termination of offensive biowarfare programs by the U.S. and the Soviet Union.

Section 5: Contemporary Concerns and Rogue States

Despite international agreements, concerns over biowarfare persist into the 21st century. Rogue states like North Korea have been suspected of maintaining active bioweapons programs, raising fears of a resurgence in biowarfare research. The threat of bioterrorism has also gained prominence, with terrorist organizations seeking to exploit advances in biotechnology for malevolent purposes.

Section 6: Ethical Dilemmas and Lessons Learned

The history of 20th-century biowarfare programs raises profound ethical dilemmas. Scientists and policymakers faced moral questions about the use of their knowledge for destructive purposes. These programs also underscore the need for vigilance, international cooperation, and strong regulations to prevent the misuse of biological research.

In conclusion, the 20th century witnessed the rise and fall of biowarfare programs on a global scale. From the dark experiments of Unit 731 to the termination of offensive programs by major powers, this period is a stark reminder of the dual-use nature of scientific knowledge. The lessons learned from this history should guide us in the 21st century as we navigate the ever-evolving landscape of biotechnology and security.

This overview provides a glimpse into the complex and troubling history of 20th-century biowarfare programs. If you would like more information on any specific aspect or if you have any further questions, please let me know.

World War I (1914-1918)

Causes:

World War I, often referred to as the Great War, was a global conflict that originated in Europe. Its causes can be traced to a complex web of factors, including:

1.   Nationalism: Intense pride and loyalty to one's nation led to tensions, especially in the Balkans.
2.   Imperialism: European powers competed for colonies and resources, leading to rivalries.
3.   Militarism: An arms race between major powers escalated tensions.
4.   Alliance System: Entangling alliances like the Triple Entente (France, Russia, Britain) and the Triple Alliance (Germany, Austria-Hungary, Italy) turned local conflicts into a global war.

Key Events:

1.   Assassination of Archduke Franz Ferdinand (June 28, 1914): The assassination in Sarajevo, Bosnia, by a Serbian nationalist triggered the war.
2.   Declaration of War: Austria-Hungary declared war on Serbia, leading to a chain reaction of declarations across Europe.
3.   Western Front: Stalemate and trench warfare characterized the Western Front.
4.   Eastern Front: Fierce battles between Germany, Austria-Hungary, and Russia occurred.
5.   US Involvement: The sinking of the RMS Lusitania and the Zimmermann Telegram prompted the United States to join the Allies in 1917.
6.   1918: Turning Point: Allied offensives and the collapse of Central Powers led to an armistice on November 11, 1918.

Consequences:

1.   Treaty of Versailles (1919): Imposed harsh terms on Germany, leading to resentment and economic hardship.
2.   League of Nations: Established to prevent future conflicts but faced challenges in its effectiveness.
3.   Redrawing of Maps: New nations were created, and empires dissolved.
4.   Economic Impact: War debts and reparations strained economies worldwide.
5.   Precursor to World War II: Unresolved issues sowed the seeds for the next global conflict.

World War II (1939-1945)

Causes:

World War II was a continuation of tensions from World War I, exacerbated by several factors:

1.   Treaty of Versailles: The punitive terms on Germany created instability in Europe.
2.   Rise of Totalitarian Regimes: Adolf Hitler's Nazi Germany, Benito Mussolini's Fascist Italy, and expansionist Japan pursued aggressive policies.
3.   Appeasement: Western powers initially adopted a policy of appeasement, hoping to avoid another war.
4.   Invasion of Poland (1939): Germany's invasion prompted Britain and France to declare war, marking the start of WWII.

Key Events:

1.   Blitzkrieg: Germany's rapid conquests of Poland, France, and other nations in Europe.
2.   Battle of Britain (1940): The Royal Air Force's successful defense against the German Luftwaffe.
3.   Operation Barbarossa (1941): Hitler's invasion of the Soviet Union.
4.   Pearl Harbor (1941): Japan's attack on the U.S. led to American entry into the war.
5.   D-Day (1944): Allied invasion of Normandy marked the beginning of the liberation of Western Europe.
6.   Atomic Bombs: The U.S. dropped atomic bombs on Hiroshima and Nagasaki, leading to Japan's surrender in 1945.

Consequences:

1.   The Holocaust: The systematic genocide of six million Jews by Nazi Germany.
2.   United Nations: Formed in 1945 to promote peace and cooperation.
3.   Nuremberg Trials: Nazi war criminals were tried for crimes against humanity.
4.   Cold War: Tensions between the U.S. and the Soviet Union emerged, leading to decades of rivalry.
5.   Decolonization: European empires crumbled, and many nations gained independence.
6.   Reconstruction: Europe and Asia faced widespread devastation, requiring massive rebuilding efforts.

In summary, World War I and World War II were two of the most significant conflicts in human history. While World War I stemmed from complex factors and ended with the Treaty of Versailles, World War II was driven by the aggressive expansion of totalitarian regimes and ended with the use of atomic weapons. Both wars had profound and lasting effects on the world, shaping the course of the 20th century and beyond.

The Cold War Bioweapons Programs: A Silent and Deadly Struggle

The Cold War was a period of intense ideological conflict and military buildup between the United States and the Soviet Union, lasting roughly from the end of World War II in 1945 to the early 1990s. While the arms race and the threat of nuclear war are often at the forefront of discussions about this era, there is another, more insidious aspect of the Cold War that often goes overlooked: bioweapons programs.

During the Cold War, both superpowers engaged in extensive research and development of biological weapons. These programs, shrouded in secrecy, posed a different kind of threat compared to the better-known nuclear arms race. Biological weapons were considered by many to be the "poor man's atomic bomb" due to their potentially catastrophic effects and relative ease of production. This essay explores the history, motivations, and consequences of Cold War bioweapons programs, shedding light on this hidden chapter of the Cold War.

I. The Origins of Cold War Bioweapons Programs

To understand the development of bioweapons programs during the Cold War, it's essential to trace their origins. The roots of biowarfare can be found in the use of biological agents in earlier conflicts, such as the deliberate spread of smallpox-infected blankets by British forces during the French and Indian War. However, the scale and sophistication of these programs expanded significantly during World War II.

A. Japanese Bioweapons in World War II

One of the earliest examples of state-sponsored bioweapons research can be found in Imperial Japan. Unit 731, led by the infamous Shiro Ishii, conducted extensive experiments on humans, animals, and pathogens during World War II. These experiments aimed to develop biological weapons for potential use against Allied forces. Ishii's unit engaged in some of the most heinous acts of biological warfare, including the dissemination of plague-infected fleas over Chinese cities, resulting in the deaths of thousands.

The U.S. government, aware of the Japanese program, offered immunity to Ishii and his researchers in exchange for their data. This controversial decision laid the foundation for America's own bioweapons research in the post-war era.

B. The Emergence of Bioweapons Research in the United States

Following World War II, the United States initiated its bioweapons program under the code name "Operation Paperclip." This program recruited former Nazi scientists, including those involved in biological warfare research, to bolster American expertise in the field. Dr. Erich Traub, a renowned virologist who had worked on the Nazi bioweapons program, was one such recruit. He played a pivotal role in establishing the U.S. bioweapons program, which was primarily based at Fort Detrick in Maryland.

The United States' interest in bioweapons was driven by several factors. First, there was a genuine fear that the Soviet Union might develop a biological arsenal, prompting the U.S. to maintain parity. Second, bioweapons were seen as a more cost-effective and politically palatable option compared to nuclear weapons. Finally, the secrecy surrounding bioweapons research allowed for plausible deniability in the event of an attack.

II. The Soviet Union's Bioweapons Program

The Soviet Union, too, embarked on an ambitious bioweapons program during the Cold War. While details of this program remained hidden for many years, information began to surface following the dissolution of the Soviet Union in the early 1990s.

A. The Soviet Bioweapons Program's Scale and Scope

Soviet bioweapons efforts were vast and comprehensive, involving multiple research institutes and facilities across the country. One of the most notorious was Vector Institute, located in Siberia. The program, like its American counterpart, drew on the expertise of former Nazi scientists and conducted research on a wide range of pathogens.

Notably, the Soviet Union pursued research into "designer diseases" – pathogens engineered for specific targets or vulnerabilities. This included efforts to create antibiotic-resistant strains of bacteria and viruses. The extent of these projects showcased the USSR's commitment to bioweapons as a strategic asset.

B. The Sverdlovsk Anthrax Incident

The secrecy surrounding the Soviet bioweapons program was punctuated by a tragic accident in 1979. In the city of Sverdlovsk (now Yekaterinburg), an accidental release of anthrax spores from a Soviet bioweapons facility led to a local outbreak. The Soviet government initially denied any wrongdoing and attributed the outbreak to contaminated meat. However, evidence later revealed the true nature of the incident.

The Sverdlovsk anthrax incident provided a rare glimpse into the Soviet bioweapons program's activities. It also underscored the dangers of conducting research on deadly pathogens in secret, as the incident resulted in the deaths of at least 64 people.

III. Biological Weapons Convention and International Efforts

Amid growing concerns about the proliferation of bioweapons during the Cold War, international efforts were made to curtail their development and use.

A. Biological Weapons Convention (BWC)

In 1972, the Biological Weapons Convention was signed, banning the development, production, and stockpiling of biological weapons. The BWC aimed to prevent the use of biological agents as weapons of war and promote peaceful cooperation in the field of biology. Both the United States and the Soviet Union were signatories to the treaty.

However, enforcing the BWC was challenging due to the secretive nature of bioweapons programs. Verification measures were limited, and allegations of non-compliance were difficult to substantiate. The BWC relied on self-reporting and trust among nations, making it inherently vulnerable to violations.

B. Allegations of Violations

Throughout the Cold War, allegations of bioweapons violations were not uncommon. Both the United States and the Soviet Union were accused of breaching the BWC, but concrete evidence was often elusive.

One notable case involved the United States' development of the bioweapon known as "Agent Orange" during the Vietnam War. While primarily used as a defoliant, Agent Orange had severe health consequences for both American soldiers and Vietnamese civilians. Some argued that its effects constituted a violation of the BWC.

Similarly, the Soviet Union faced allegations of using biological agents during the Afghanistan conflict in the 1980s. The use of mycotoxins, toxins produced by fungi, was suspected in the Afghan war. However, conclusive evidence remained elusive.

IV. The Legacy of Cold War Bioweapons Programs

As the Cold War drew to a close in the early 1990s, both the United States and the Soviet Union officially declared an end to their offensive bioweapons programs. The dissolution of the Soviet Union allowed for greater transparency regarding its bioweapons activities, with former Soviet scientists providing valuable insights into the program's scale and objectives.

A. The Collapse of the Soviet Bioweapons Program

The unraveling of the Soviet bioweapons program revealed its staggering size and ambition. It became evident that the Soviet Union had developed an extensive arsenal of biological weapons, including deadly pathogens such as smallpox, anthrax, and plague. This revelation raised concerns about the security of these materials following the Soviet Union's collapse.

Efforts were made to secure and eliminate biological weapons stockpiles, but the process was complicated by economic turmoil and the redirection of resources in post-Soviet Russia. Concerns about "brain drain" – the emigration of talented scientists – also emerged, as many researchers faced economic hardship in the wake of the Soviet Union's disintegration. To address these concerns, various international programs, including the Cooperative Threat Reduction (CTR) program initiated by the United States, aimed to support the redirection of former Soviet bioweapons experts towards peaceful scientific endeavors.

B. The United States' Decision to Dismantle its Bioweapons Program

In the United States, the end of the Cold War prompted a reevaluation of the bioweapons program's necessity. Concerns about the ethical implications of bioweapons research and the potential for accidental releases led to a significant shift in policy. In 1969, President Richard Nixon unilaterally renounced the use of biological weapons and ordered the destruction of existing stockpiles.

The United States took further steps towards transparency and disarmament by formally ending its offensive bioweapons program in 1972. This decision was influenced by the Biological Weapons Convention (BWC), which the U.S. had ratified the same year. However, the country continued to maintain a robust defensive bioweapons program, focusing on research to counteract potential bioweapons threats.

C. Contemporary Concerns and the Dual-Use Dilemma

While the Cold War-era bioweapons programs of the United States and the Soviet Union officially ended, concerns about biological weapons have not disappeared. The dual-use dilemma persists, wherein scientific advancements that can be used for both peaceful and nefarious purposes create challenges for biosecurity.

One example is the field of synthetic biology, which enables the creation of custom-designed organisms and pathogens. While this technology has immense potential for medicine and biotechnology, it also raises concerns about bioterrorism and the accidental release of engineered pathogens.

The 2001 anthrax attacks in the United States highlighted the continued relevance of bioweapons concerns. Letters containing anthrax spores were mailed to several individuals, leading to multiple deaths and widespread fear. The incident demonstrated the vulnerability of modern societies to bioterrorism and the need for robust public health responses.

V. Contemporary Bioweapons Threats and Global Preparedness

As we move further into the 21st century, the threat of bioweapons has not diminished. In fact, advances in biotechnology and the globalization of scientific knowledge have made it easier for both state and non-state actors to acquire the expertise and materials necessary for bioweapons development.

A. State-Sponsored Bioweapons Programs

Several countries, including North Korea, Iran, and Syria, have been suspected of maintaining or pursuing bioweapons programs in violation of the Biological Weapons Convention. These suspicions are difficult to confirm due to the clandestine nature of such programs. Nevertheless, they underscore the ongoing relevance of bioweapons as a security concern.

B. Non-State Actors and Bioterrorism

The threat of bioterrorism has also grown in prominence. Non-state actors, such as terrorist organizations, have expressed interest in bioweapons. While conducting large-scale bioweapons attacks is technically challenging, even a small-scale attack with a deadly pathogen could have devastating consequences.

Global preparedness for bioweapons threats has improved in recent years. International organizations, such as the World Health Organization (WHO) and the Centers for Disease Control and Prevention (CDC), work to monitor and respond to infectious disease outbreaks. The Global Health Security Agenda (GHSA) seeks to enhance international collaboration on biosecurity and biopreparedness.

VI. The Ongoing Challenge of Bioweapons

The history of Cold War bioweapons programs serves as a sobering reminder of the human capacity for both scientific achievement and destructive intent. The pursuit of bioweapons during that era led to horrific experiments, accidental outbreaks, and ethical dilemmas. The legacy of these programs continues to shape our approach to biotechnology and biosecurity today.

In the post-Cold War era, international efforts have been made to prevent the use of biological weapons through treaties like the Biological Weapons Convention. However, the persistent threat of bioterrorism, state-sponsored programs, and the dual-use dilemma mean that vigilance is still necessary.

The key to addressing the ongoing challenge of bioweapons lies in continued international cooperation, transparency, and the responsible use of biotechnology. As science advances, it is essential to strike a balance between harnessing its potential for the betterment of humanity and guarding against its misuse for destructive purposes.

Ultimately, the story of Cold War bioweapons programs serves as a stark reminder that the pursuit of knowledge and power can lead down dark and dangerous paths. In an increasingly interconnected and biologically advanced world, the lessons of history must guide our efforts to prevent the catastrophic consequences of bioweapons.

Modern Bioweapon Threats

In the ever-evolving landscape of global security threats, bioweapons have emerged as a significant concern. Modern bioweapon threats pose unique challenges that demand a deep understanding of biology, technology, and international relations. This comprehensive overview explores the nature of these threats, their potential consequences, the actors involved, and the efforts being made to mitigate them.

I. Understanding Bioweapons

1.1 Definition of Bioweapons

Bioweapons, short for biological weapons, are agents derived from living organisms, such as bacteria, viruses, and toxins, that are intentionally used to harm or kill people, animals, or plants. Unlike conventional weapons, bioweapons harness the power of biology, making them invisible, hard to detect, and potentially devastating.

1.2 Historical Perspective

The use of bioweapons dates back centuries, with documented instances of poisoned arrows in ancient warfare. However, modern bioweapon development began in the 20th century, with notable examples including the use of anthrax by Japan during World War II and the Soviet Union's extensive bioweapons program during the Cold War.

II. Modern Bioweapon Threat Agents

2.1 Pathogens

Pathogens are the primary agents used in bioweapons. These can include bacteria, viruses, and fungi. Notable examples include anthrax (Bacillus anthracis), smallpox (Variola virus), and botulinum toxin (Clostridium botulinum).

2.2 Genetic Engineering

Advances in genetic engineering have made it possible to modify pathogens for specific purposes. This includes enhancing their virulence, increasing resistance to treatments, or even designing entirely synthetic organisms. Such modifications raise concerns about the creation of superbugs or designer bioweapons.

2.3 Dual-Use Research

Many scientific advancements that can improve public health can also be applied to bioweapons. Dual-use research refers to studies with both beneficial and harmful applications. Striking a balance between scientific progress and security is a significant challenge.

III. Actors in the Bioweapon Threat Landscape

3.1 State Actors

Several countries have been known to develop bioweapons or maintain bioweapon research programs. Historically, the United States, Russia, China, and North Korea have been associated with state-sponsored bioweapon programs. The Biological Weapons Convention (BWC) prohibits the use of bioweapons, but verifying compliance remains a challenge.

3.2 Non-State Actors

Terrorist organizations and criminal networks have shown interest in bioweapons. The lack of a return address and their potential for mass casualties make bioweapons attractive to these groups. The Aum Shinrikyo cult's attempted use of sarin gas in the 1990s exemplifies this threat.

IV. Modern Challenges in Bioweapon Threats

4.1 Rapid Advancements in Biotechnology

The biotechnology revolution has democratized access to tools and knowledge needed for bioweapon development. This raises concerns about the ability of non-state actors or rogue individuals to create and deploy bioweapons.

4.2 Cyber-Bio Convergence

The convergence of cyber and biological threats, known as cyber-bio threats, poses unique challenges. Cyberattacks can disrupt biological research, manipulate data, or even control lab equipment, potentially leading to accidental or deliberate release of dangerous pathogens.

4.3 Pandemic Preparedness

The COVID-19 pandemic has exposed vulnerabilities in global pandemic preparedness and response. A deliberate release of a bioweapon could trigger a similar crisis, underscoring the need for improved surveillance, early warning systems, and international cooperation.

V. Potential Consequences of Bioweapon Attacks

5.1 Human Casualties

Bioweapon attacks have the potential to cause significant human casualties. Highly contagious pathogens could spread rapidly, overwhelming healthcare systems and causing mass fatalities.

5.2 Economic Disruption

A bioweapon attack could disrupt critical infrastructure, supply chains, and economies. The economic consequences of a large-scale bioweapon incident would likely be severe and long-lasting.

5.3 Psychological Impact

Bioweapons not only harm physical health but also have a profound psychological impact. Fear, uncertainty, and social disruption can lead to long-term psychological trauma.

VI. International Response and Legal Frameworks

6.1 Biological Weapons Convention (BWC)

The BWC is the primary international treaty aimed at preventing the use of biological weapons. It prohibits the development, production, and acquisition of bioweapons. However, enforcement and verification remain challenging.

6.2 United Nations Security Council Resolution 1540

This resolution obligates member states to take measures to prevent non-state actors from acquiring weapons of mass destruction, including bioweapons. It emphasizes the importance of securing biological materials and strengthening national controls.

6.3 National Biodefense Strategies

Many countries have developed national biodefense strategies to address the bioweapon threat. These strategies include measures to enhance biosurveillance, improve response capabilities, and secure biological research facilities.

VII. Mitigating Modern Bioweapon Threats

7.1 Strengthening Biosurveillance

Early detection is crucial in containing a bioweapon threat. Advanced biosurveillance systems can monitor for unusual disease patterns and rapidly identify potential bioweapon outbreaks.

7.2 International Collaboration

Addressing bioweapon threats requires international cooperation. Countries must share information, expertise, and resources to respond effectively to bioweapon incidents.

7.3 Biosecurity Measures

Securing biological research facilities and regulating access to dangerous pathogens are critical components of bioweapon threat mitigation. Stringent biosecurity measures can reduce the risk of accidental or intentional release.

VIII. Future Trends and Challenges

8.1 Synthetic Biology

Advances in synthetic biology have the potential to revolutionize bioweapon development. The ability to design and engineer organisms from scratch presents new challenges for security and oversight.

8.2 Ethical Considerations

The ethical implications of bioweapon research and development are complex. Striking a balance between scientific progress and security while upholding ethical principles is an ongoing challenge.

8.3 Emerging Diseases

The continued emergence of new infectious diseases, such as Zika and Ebola, highlights the importance of preparedness for bioweapon threats. Lessons from natural outbreaks can inform bioweapon response strategies.

Modern bioweapon threats represent a complex and evolving challenge. The potential consequences of a bioweapon attack are severe, affecting not only human lives but also economies and societies. Addressing this threat requires a multi-faceted approach, including international cooperation, improved biosurveillance, and robust biosecurity measures. As biotechnology continues to advance, vigilance and preparedness are paramount in safeguarding global security against bioweapon threats.

State-Sponsored Biological Warfare: A Looming Threat to Global Security

In an ever-evolving world of warfare, the use of biological agents as tools of destruction has emerged as a chilling and potentially catastrophic threat. State-sponsored biological warfare, the deliberate manipulation and deployment of pathogens and toxins by governments, poses a grave danger to global security. While the use of biological agents in warfare is not a new concept, recent advancements in biotechnology and our interconnected global society have amplified the risks associated with such weapons. This essay delves into the ominous realm of state-sponsored biological warfare, examining its history, the motivations behind it, its potential consequences, and the measures required to prevent its catastrophic effects.

1.   Historical Perspective

The history of biological warfare dates back centuries, with accounts of its use as early as 1346 when Mongol forces reportedly catapulted plague-infected corpses into the Crimean city of Kaffa. However, it was during the 20th century that state-sponsored biological warfare programs gained prominence. Notably, during World War II, Japan's Unit 731 conducted gruesome experiments on humans and developed biological weapons, including anthrax and plague, which they deployed against Chinese cities.

Following World War II, the United States and the Soviet Union engaged in a biological arms race, developing and stockpiling a wide range of biological agents. The Biological Weapons Convention (BWC) of 1972 sought to curb the proliferation of such weapons, banning their development, production, and acquisition. Nevertheless, covert state-sponsored programs continued in several countries, creating an atmosphere of suspicion and insecurity.

2.   Motivations Behind State-Sponsored Biological Warfare

Understanding the motivations behind state-sponsored biological warfare is crucial to developing effective countermeasures. Several factors drive nations to explore and maintain biological weapons capabilities:

2.1. Strategic Deterrence

Biological weapons can serve as a form of deterrence. The possession of these weapons can dissuade potential adversaries from military aggression, fearing the unpredictable and devastating consequences of a biological attack.

2.2. Covert Warfare

Biological agents can be used in covert operations, allowing states to wage low-intensity conflicts without overtly declaring war. This provides a level of deniability and complicates attribution.

2.3. Asymmetric Warfare

Biological weapons can level the playing field for nations with limited military capabilities, enabling them to inflict significant harm on technologically superior adversaries.

2.4. Biotechnology Advancements

Advancements in biotechnology have made it easier to manipulate and engineer biological agents, reducing the barriers to entry for states seeking to develop these weapons.

3.   Potential Consequences of State-Sponsored Biological Warfare

The consequences of state-sponsored biological warfare are nothing short of catastrophic, encompassing a range of immediate and long-term impacts on society, the environment, and international relations.

3.1. Loss of Human Life

Biological weapons have the potential to cause mass casualties. A well-coordinated biological attack on a densely populated area could result in the deaths of thousands, or even millions, of people.

3.2. Economic Disruption

The aftermath of a biological attack can severely disrupt economies. The need for medical care, quarantine measures, and the fear of further infection can lead to a collapse in trade, tourism, and productivity.

3.3. Societal Chaos

The fear and panic resulting from a biological attack can lead to societal chaos. Mass migrations, breakdowns in law and order, and civil unrest can further exacerbate the crisis.

3.4. Environmental Damage

Biological agents released into the environment can have lasting ecological effects. Pathogens can infect wildlife, disrupt ecosystems, and lead to long-term environmental damage.

3.5. International Relations

State-sponsored biological warfare can trigger international conflicts, erode trust between nations, and undermine diplomatic efforts. The use of biological weapons can lead to retaliation and escalation.

4.   Challenges in Detection and Attribution

Detecting and attributing a biological attack to a specific state actor is a complex and challenging task. Unlike conventional weapons, which leave physical evidence, biological agents can be difficult to trace back to their source. The following challenges hinder effective detection and attribution:

4.1. Dual-Use Facilities

Biological research facilities often have legitimate civilian applications, making it difficult to distinguish between research for defensive purposes and the development of offensive biological weapons.

4.2. Deniability

State-sponsored biological warfare often involves covert operations and plausible deniability, making it challenging to prove a nation's involvement.

4.3. Rapid Spread

Biological agents can spread rapidly, complicating efforts to trace their origins. This can lead to delays in identifying the source of an outbreak.

4.4. Evolving Threat Landscape

Advancements in biotechnology enable the creation of genetically modified agents that may not match known pathogens, making detection even more challenging.

5.   Preventive Measures

Preventing state-sponsored biological warfare requires a multi-faceted approach involving international cooperation, diplomacy, and robust safeguards:

5.1. Strengthening the Biological Weapons Convention (BWC)

The BWC should be reinforced with stricter verification mechanisms, transparency measures, and penalties for non-compliance. Additionally, efforts to promote universal adherence to the treaty should be intensified.

5.2. Promoting Transparency

States should openly share information about their biodefense programs and facilities, reducing suspicions and fostering trust among nations.

5.3. International Monitoring

International organizations and agencies should be empowered to monitor and inspect biotechnology facilities to ensure compliance with the BWC.

5.4. Biotechnology Regulations

Stringent regulations on the handling and transfer of dangerous pathogens and genetic engineering technologies should be implemented globally.

5.5. Preparedness and Response

Nations should invest in robust public health infrastructure and emergency response systems to mitigate the impact of biological attacks.

6.   Case Studies

Several countries have been accused of or suspected of engaging in state-sponsored biological warfare activities. Two notable examples are:

6.1. The Soviet Union

The Soviet Union maintained an extensive biological weapons program during the Cold War. This program, known as Biopreparat, produced a variety of deadly agents, including anthrax, smallpox, and tularemia. While the program was officially terminated in 1992, there are concerns about the security of the remaining stockpiles.

6.2. North Korea

North Korea has been accused of developing biological weapons alongside its nuclear program. The secretive nature of the regime makes it challenging to assess the extent of its biological weapons capabilities.

7. The Role of Biotechnology

Advancements in biotechnology have dual-use applications, enabling both beneficial scientific research and the development of biological weapons. To address this challenge, the international community must strike a delicate balance between promoting scientific progress and preventing its misuse:

7.1. Dual-Use Research Oversight

Research institutions should implement strict oversight of dual-use research projects, ensuring that the potential risks and benefits are carefully considered.

7.2. Education and Awareness

Scientists should be educated about the ethical implications of their work, and awareness campaigns should be conducted to highlight the dangers of biological warfare.

7.3. Export Controls

Governments should establish export controls on equipment, materials, and technologies that can be used in the development of biological weapons.

State-sponsored biological warfare represents one of the most menacing threats to global security. The potential consequences of a biological attack are staggering, encompassing loss of life, economic disruption, societal chaos, environmental damage, and strained international relations. To prevent such a catastrophe, nations must work together to strengthen the Biological Weapons Convention, promote transparency,and implement rigorous monitoring and regulatory measures. It is imperative that the international community takes proactive steps to prevent the development, production, and use of biological weapons by state actors.

In addition to these measures, there must be a renewed commitment to disarmament and the peaceful use of biotechnology. This includes fostering a culture of responsible research, with scientists and institutions taking into account the ethical considerations of their work. Raising awareness about the risks associated with biological warfare is also crucial, as an informed public can advocate for effective policies and hold governments accountable.

Furthermore, it is essential for countries to invest in their public health infrastructure and emergency response capabilities. A strong and agile healthcare system can mitigate the impact of a biological attack, providing timely medical care, quarantine measures, and vaccination campaigns.

The examples of the Soviet Union and North Korea underscore the ongoing challenges of monitoring and verifying compliance with disarmament treaties. In a world where rogue states and non-state actors seek to acquire biological weapons, intelligence sharing and international cooperation become paramount. Nations must be vigilant and ready to respond collectively to any indication of biological weapons development.

Ultimately, the prevention of state-sponsored biological warfare is not solely the responsibility of governments but of the entire global community. It requires a concerted effort, with nations setting aside their differences in the pursuit of a safer and more secure world. The devastating consequences of biological warfare should serve as a stark reminder of the urgent need for action.

In conclusion, state-sponsored biological warfare represents a dark and perilous threat to humanity. The historical context, motivations, and potential consequences of such warfare demand our attention and vigilance. Preventing the use of biological weapons requires international cooperation, transparency, and a commitment to disarmament. The world must unite to ensure that the specter of state-sponsored biological warfare remains in the realm of history, rather than becoming a haunting reality for future generations.

Notable Offenders in Biological Warfare

Biological warfare, the use of living organisms or their byproducts as weapons of war, has a dark and disturbing history. Throughout the centuries, nations and individuals have explored the use of pathogens, toxins, and other biological agents to harm and incapacitate their enemies. This article explores notable offenders in the realm of biological warfare, highlighting key historical instances and the consequences of these actions.

The use of biological agents as weapons is not a recent phenomenon. Historical records dating back to antiquity document instances of poisoned arrows and contaminated water supplies used in warfare. However, the modern era saw a more systematic and widespread pursuit of biological warfare capabilities, often with dire consequences.

1. Ancient and Medieval Practices

Before delving into the modern era, it's essential to recognize that biological warfare was not exclusive to contemporary times. Ancient and medieval societies employed various tactics, often rudimentary, to infect their adversaries. For instance:

a. The Siege of Caffa (1346)

During the Mongol siege of the Crimean city of Caffa, corpses of plague victims were catapulted over the city walls. This is believed to have contributed to the spread of the Black Death in Europe.

2. The Modern Era

The 20th century marked a significant shift in the development and deployment of biological weapons. Notable offenders during this period include state actors, terrorist groups, and individuals driven by ideological or political motives.

a. Japan's Unit 731

One of the most infamous perpetrators of biological warfare during World War II was Unit 731, a covert biological and chemical warfare research and development unit of the Imperial Japanese Army. Led by General Shiro Ishii, Unit 731 conducted horrific experiments on live human subjects and unleashed deadly pathogens on Chinese cities. The extent of their atrocities was vast, and their actions resulted in thousands of deaths.

b. The United States and Fort Detrick

During the Cold War, the United States invested heavily in biological warfare research. Fort Detrick, located in Maryland, was at the forefront of these efforts. The U.S. Army conducted experiments involving biological agents, such as anthrax and Q fever, to assess their potential as weapons. The program was eventually terminated in 1969 due to international agreements, but it left a dark mark on U.S. history.

c. The Soviet Union's Biopreparat

The Soviet Union's Biopreparat was a secretive bioweapons program that operated during the Cold War. It had multiple research and production facilities dedicated to developing deadly pathogens. Notably, an accidental release of anthrax spores in Sverdlovsk in 1979 resulted in at least 66 deaths. The Soviet Union's extensive biological warfare program only came to light after its dissolution.

d. Aum Shinrikyo's Sarin Gas Attack

Although primarily known for its use of chemical weapons, the Japanese cult Aum Shinrikyo also attempted to deploy biological agents. In 1993, they released botulinum toxin in Tokyo, but the attack failed to cause significant harm. This incident revealed the group's intention to use biological warfare as part of its apocalyptic ideology.

3. The Biological Weapons Convention

Recognizing the grave threat posed by biological weapons, the international community took steps to curb their proliferation. The Biological Weapons Convention (BWC), which came into force in 1975, was a landmark agreement that prohibited the development, production, and acquisition of biological weapons. However, enforcement remains challenging, and there have been allegations of non-compliance.

a. The Iraq Case

Iraq's violation of the BWC gained significant attention during the 1990s. After the Gulf War, it was revealed that Saddam Hussein's regime had a clandestine biological weapons program. Inspectors from the United Nations Special Commission (UNSCOM) uncovered evidence of Iraq's efforts to weaponize anthrax and other pathogens. This led to extensive inspections and disarmament efforts, ultimately culminating in the U.S.-led invasion of Iraq in 2003.

4. Contemporary Concerns

Biological warfare remains a grave concern in the 21st century. Notable offenders include states suspected of maintaining or developing biological weapons programs, as well as the potential threat posed by non-state actors.

a. North Korea

North Korea has long been suspected of pursuing biological weapons as part of its overall military strategy. Limited information is available due to the secretive nature of the regime, but reports suggest that North Korea possesses the capacity to produce and weaponize biological agents.

b. The Syrian Civil War

The Syrian Civil War, which began in 2011, raised concerns about the use of chemical and biological weapons. There have been allegations of chemical and biological attacks, though verifying these claims amidst the chaos of the conflict has been challenging. The use of such weapons, if confirmed, would constitute a grave violation of international norms.

c. Bioterrorism Threat

In addition to state actors, the threat of bioterrorism looms large. Terrorist organizations and individuals with access to biotechnological knowledge could potentially engineer and deploy biological agents. Efforts to prevent bioterrorism include improved surveillance, international cooperation, and securing biological research facilities.

Notable offenders in biological warfare span centuries and include state actors, secretive programs, and terrorist organizations. The development and use of biological weapons have left a trail of suffering and death in their wake. The international community has made efforts to prohibit and curb the use of such weapons, exemplified by the Biological Weapons Convention. However, the threat persists in the form of state actors and the potential for bioterrorism. Vigilance, diplomacy, and adherence to international agreements remain crucial in preventing the catastrophic consequences of biological warfare.

International Agreements and Treaties on Biological Warfare

Biological warfare, often referred to as biowarfare or germ warfare, is the use of biological toxins or infectious agents, such as bacteria, viruses, and fungi, with the intent to harm or kill humans, animals, or plants. This form of warfare has a long and dark history, dating back centuries, with various instances of its use recorded throughout time. Recognizing the potential catastrophic consequences of biological weapons, the international community has come together to establish a framework of agreements and treaties aimed at preventing the development, production, and use of such weapons. This essay will delve into the history and evolution of international agreements and treaties on biological warfare, exploring their significance in maintaining global security and the challenges they face in an ever-changing world.

Historical Background

The use of biological agents as weapons is not a recent phenomenon. Historical records suggest that various civilizations employed crude forms of biological warfare, such as catapulting plague-infected corpses over city walls, as far back as the 6th century BC. However, it was during the 20th century that biological warfare reached new heights, particularly during World War I, when both Allied and Central Powers researched and attempted to deploy biological agents. Fortunately, these attempts were largely ineffective, but they underscored the need for international cooperation to address the growing threat of biological warfare.

The First International Efforts

In the aftermath of World War I, the international community recognized the need to address the threat of biological weapons. The Geneva Protocol of 1925, formally known as the Protocol for the Prohibition of the Use in War of Asphyxiating, Poisonous or Other Gases, and of Bacteriological Methods of Warfare, was a significant milestone. While it primarily focused on chemical weapons, it also included a prohibition on the use of biological agents in warfare. However, the Geneva Protocol had significant limitations; it did not ban the development, production, or stockpiling of biological agents for offensive purposes, nor did it establish mechanisms for verification and enforcement.

The Cold War Era and the Biological Weapons Convention

The post-World War II period, marked by the intensification of the Cold War, saw a proliferation of biological weapons programs. Both the United States and the Soviet

Union invested heavily in biowarfare research and development. This arms race prompted renewed efforts to address the issue of biological warfare.

The Biological Weapons Convention (BWC), which came into force in 1975, represented a significant step forward in international efforts to control biological weapons. The BWC is the first multilateral treaty to explicitly prohibit the development, production, and possession of biological weapons. Its preamble emphasizes the need to "exclude completely the possibility of bacteriological (biological) agents and toxins being used as weapons." Under the BWC, member states committed to destroying their existing biological weapon stockpiles, not developing new ones, and using biological agents only for peaceful and defensive purposes.

Despite its groundbreaking nature, the BWC has faced significant challenges. One of the main issues has been the absence of a verification and inspection regime, unlike arms control agreements related to nuclear weapons. This lack of monitoring mechanisms made it difficult to verify compliance and led to suspicions among member states.

The 1990s: A Turning Point

The 1990s witnessed a series of events that had a profound impact on international efforts to control biological weapons. Two notable incidents were pivotal in shaping the discourse on biowarfare:

1.   The End of the Cold War: The collapse of the Soviet Union in 1991 revealed the extent of its biological weapons program, which had been shrouded in secrecy for decades. The Soviet Union's admission of its offensive biowarfare program was a major turning point in international efforts to control biological weapons. This revelation underscored the importance of transparency and confidence-building measures.
2.   The Aum Shinrikyo Cult Attacks: In 1995, the Aum Shinrikyo cult carried out a sarin gas attack on the Tokyo subway system. Although not a biological attack, this incident raised concerns about non-state actors acquiring and using weapons of mass destruction, including biological agents. It highlighted the need to strengthen the BWC and develop mechanisms to prevent bioterrorism.

Strengthening the BWC

In response to these challenges, efforts were made to strengthen the BWC. The Ad Hoc Group of the States Parties to the BWC was established in 1994 to negotiate a legally binding protocol to enhance the effectiveness of the Convention. However, negotiations faced significant hurdles, and by 2001, the process had reached an impasse, leading to the collapse of the protocol negotiations.

Despite this setback, the BWC continued to evolve. States parties adopted a series of confidence-building measures (CBMs) to enhance transparency and cooperation. These CBMs included declarations of past offensive biowarfare programs, information-sharing on dual-use biotechnologies, and the establishment of national points of contact. While these measures were non-binding, they represented a step forward in building trust among member states.

The BWC also established the Implementation Support Unit (ISU) to assist states parties in implementing the Convention and to promote international cooperation in areas related to biological security. The ISU played a crucial role in facilitating dialogue and capacity-building among member states.

The 21st Century: Emerging Threats and Challenges

As the 21st century progressed, new challenges and threats related to biological warfare emerged, necessitating continued international efforts to adapt and strengthen the existing framework of agreements and treaties.

1.   Advancements in Biotechnology: Rapid advancements in biotechnology, including gene editing and synthetic biology, have made it easier to manipulate and engineer biological agents. This has raised concerns about the potential for the development of more sophisticated and deadly bioweapons by both state and non-state actors.

2.   Bioterrorism: The threat of bioterrorism remains a significant concern. Terrorist organizations and individuals with malicious intent may seek to acquire and use biological agents to cause widespread harm. The Aum Shinrikyo cult's attempted use of biological agents in the 1990s serves as a stark reminder of this threat.

3.   Dual-Use Dilemma: The dual-use nature of many biotechnologies presents a dilemma. Technologies that have legitimate scientific and medical applications can also be misused for biowarfare. Striking the right balance between promoting scientific progress and preventing misuse is a complex challenge.

4.   Lack of Universal Compliance: Not all countries are parties to the BWC, and compliance with its provisions remains uneven. The absence of universal participation and adherence weakens the Convention's effectiveness in preventing the proliferation of biological weapons.

5.   Verification and Enforcement: The lack of a robust verification and enforcement mechanism continues to be a fundamental weakness of the BWC. Unlike arms control agreements for nuclear weapons, there are no international inspectors or agencies with the authority to verify compliance with the Convention.

The Evolution of International Agreements and Treaties

In response to these emerging challenges, there have been several notable developments in international agreements and treaties related to biological warfare:

1.   The Biological Weapons Convention (BWC) Review Conferences: The BWC holds Review Conferences every five years to assess the implementation of the Convention and discuss ways to strengthen it. These conferences provide a platform for member states to exchange information and ideas on various aspects of biological security. The most recent Review Conference in 2016 led to the adoption of a final document that outlined various recommendations for enhancing the BWC's effectiveness and addressing contemporary challenges. These recommendations included measures to strengthen national implementation, enhance international cooperation, and promote transparency.

2.   United Nations Security Council Resolution 1540: Adopted in 2004, Resolution 1540 is a landmark measure that focuses on the prevention of the proliferation of weapons of mass destruction (WMDs), including biological weapons. It obliges all United Nations member states to take measures to prevent non-state actors, such as terrorist organizations, from acquiring and using WMDs. While not a treaty in itself, this resolution underscores the importance of a comprehensive approach to addressing the threat of biowarfare.

3.   Global Health Security Agenda (GHSA): Although primarily focused on improving global health security and pandemic preparedness, the GHSA recognizes the link between public health and biosecurity. It emphasizes the need for countries to strengthen their capabilities to detect, respond to, and mitigate biological threats, whether natural or intentional. The GHSA promotes international collaboration to address infectious disease outbreaks and bioterrorism.

4.   International Health Regulations (IHR): The IHR, adopted by the World Health Organization (WHO) in 2005, are a set of legally binding regulations aimed at preventing the international spread of infectious diseases. While primarily focused on public health emergencies, the IHR also have implications for biosecurity. They require countries to notify the WHO of any outbreaks of certain infectious diseases, which can help detect and respond to deliberate acts of bioterrorism.

5.   Biological Risk Reduction (BRR) Program: Some countries have established national programs to reduce the risk of accidental or deliberate release of dangerous pathogens. These programs focus on enhancing laboratory safety, security, and biosecurity measures to prevent the theft or unauthorized access to dangerous biological materials.

Challenges and Future Directions

Despite these developments, numerous challenges persist in the field of international agreements and treaties on biological warfare. Addressing these challenges is essential to ensure global security and prevent the catastrophic consequences of biowarfare.

1.   Verification and Enforcement: The absence of a robust verification and enforcement mechanism continues to hinder the effectiveness of the BWC. Establishing a system of international inspections and verification, similar to those in place for nuclear disarmament treaties, remains a complex and contentious issue. Overcoming these obstacles is essential to ensure compliance with the Convention's provisions.

2.   Universal Participation: Achieving universal participation in the BWC remains a challenge. Some countries remain outside the Convention, and efforts to encourage non-member states to join have not been entirely successful. Broader participation is essential to create a global norm against biological weapons.

3.   Emerging Technologies: The rapid advancement of biotechnology and the dual-use nature of many biotechnologies make it difficult to monitor and control potentially dangerous research. Efforts to address these challenges should balance the promotion of scientific progress with measures to prevent misuse.

4.   Bioterrorism: The threat of bioterrorism remains a significant concern. Strengthening international cooperation and intelligence sharing to detect and prevent bioterrorist activities is critical. Moreover, enhancing the preparedness and response capabilities of countries to biological threats is essential.

5.   Promoting Responsible Science: Encouraging scientists and researchers to conduct their work responsibly is crucial. Codes of conduct and ethical guidelines should be promoted to ensure that scientific advancements in biotechnology are used for peaceful and beneficial purposes.

6.   Addressing Non-State Actors: Preventing non-state actors, such as terrorist groups, from acquiring and using biological weapons is a complex challenge. International efforts should focus on improving border security, intelligence sharing, and countering the radicalization of individuals with malicious intent.

International agreements and treaties on biological warfare have come a long way since the adoption of the Geneva Protocol in 1925. The Biological Weapons Convention (BWC) represents a significant achievement in prohibiting the use of biological weapons and promoting transparency and cooperation among member states. However, the evolving nature of biological threats, including emerging technologies and the potential for bioterrorism, requires ongoing adaptation and strengthening of the existing framework.

The challenges of verifying compliance, achieving universal participation, and addressing dual-use biotechnologies remain formidable. Nevertheless, international efforts, including Review Conferences, confidence-building measures, and initiatives like UN Security Council Resolution 1540, demonstrate a commitment to addressing these challenges.

In an interconnected world where the consequences of a biological attack could be devastating, international cooperation and vigilance are paramount. Strengthening the global norm against biological weapons, promoting responsible science, and enhancing biosecurity measures are all essential steps toward preventing the use of biological agents for destructive purposes. Ultimately, the goal is to ensure that advances in biotechnology are harnessed for the betterment of humanity rather than for its destruction.

Non-State Actors and Terrorism

The phenomenon of terrorism has evolved significantly in recent decades, with non-state actors playing a prominent role in its proliferation. Non-state actors, such as terrorist organizations, insurgent groups, and transnational criminal networks, have become major players on the global stage, challenging the traditional state-centric model of conflict. This essay explores the complex relationship between non-state actors and terrorism, delving into their motivations, tactics, and the challenges they pose to international security.

Defining Non-State Actors

Non-state actors encompass a diverse array of groups that operate independently of recognized states. They include terrorist organizations, insurgent groups, criminal organizations, and even non-governmental organizations (NGOs) in certain contexts. This essay primarily focuses on non-state actors involved in terrorism.

1.   Motivations of Non-State Actors

Understanding the motivations of non-state actors is crucial to grasping the root causes of terrorism. Several factors drive these groups to engage in acts of terror:

1.1 Political Goals: Many non-state actors aim to achieve political objectives, such as gaining independence, establishing a separate state, or overthrowing a government. For example, the Kurdistan Workers' Party (PKK) seeks autonomy for the Kurdish population in Turkey.

1.2 Ideological Beliefs: Ideology often plays a central role in motivating non-state actors. Groups like Al-Qaeda are driven by extremist religious ideologies, while leftist or right-wing extremist organizations may pursue their goals based on political ideologies.

1.3 Economic Gains: Some non-state actors engage in terrorism for financial reasons. Criminal organizations like drug cartels use violence and intimidation to protect their interests and expand their operations.

1.4 Revenge and Retaliation: Acts of terrorism can also be driven by a desire for revenge or retaliation against perceived injustices. The Tamil Tigers in Sri Lanka engaged in a brutal campaign of terror in response to government actions against the Tamil minority.

2.   Tactics Employed by Non-State Actors

Non-state actors employ a wide range of tactics to achieve their goals, often using terrorism as a means to an end:

2.1 Suicide Attacks: Suicide bombings have become a hallmark of many terrorist organizations, including Hamas and ISIS. These attacks are designed to instill fear and maximize casualties.

2.2 Kidnappings: Non-state actors often use kidnappings as a tactic to pressure governments or organizations into meeting their demands. The kidnapping of schoolgirls by Boko Haram in Nigeria is a notable example.

2.3 Guerrilla Warfare: Insurgent groups frequently employ guerrilla warfare tactics, blending in with the civilian population and launching hit-and-run attacks on military and government targets.

2.4 Cyberterrorism: In the digital age, non-state actors have also embraced cyberterrorism, using technology to disrupt critical infrastructure and steal sensitive information.

2.5 Propaganda and Media: Many non-state actors utilize propaganda and media campaigns to recruit supporters and spread their messages globally, leveraging social media and online platforms.

3.   Challenges Posed by Non-State Actors

Non-state actors engaged in terrorism present significant challenges to international security and governance:

3.1 Asymmetry of Power: Non-state actors often lack the military and economic resources of states, making them difficult to combat through traditional means.

3.2 Transnational Nature: Many non-state actors operate across borders, making it challenging for states to coordinate efforts to combat them effectively.

3.3 Difficulties in Attribution: Identifying the responsible parties behind terrorist attacks can be challenging, as they often operate clandestinely.

3.4 Funding and Financing: Non-state actors require funding to sustain their operations, and they often engage in illegal activities like drug trafficking or extortion to finance their activities.

3.5 Radicalization and Recruitment: Non-state actors rely on the recruitment of individuals, which can occur both locally and internationally, facilitated by online radicalization efforts.

4.   Responses to Non-State Actor Terrorism

Efforts to counter non-state actor terrorism involve a combination of military, diplomatic, and socio-economic measures:

4.1 Military Action: States often use military force to disrupt non-state actor operations. This may involve targeted drone strikes, special operations, or large-scale military campaigns.

4.2 Diplomacy and Negotiation: In some cases, states engage in negotiations with non-state actors to address their grievances and seek peaceful resolutions to conflicts.

4.3 Intelligence and Counterterrorism Cooperation: International cooperation is essential in sharing intelligence and coordinating efforts to combat terrorism.

4.4 Counterterrorism Legislation: Many states have enacted counterterrorism laws to identify, track, and prosecute individuals and groups involved in terrorism.

4.5 Countering Radicalization: Efforts to counter the radicalization of individuals often involve programs focused on education, community engagement, and addressing the root causes of extremism.

5.   Case Studies

To illustrate the complex dynamics between non-state actors and terrorism, let's examine two prominent case studies:

5.1 Al-Qaeda: Founded by Osama bin Laden in the late 1980s, Al-Qaeda became infamous for its role in the 9/11 attacks in the United States. Al-Qaeda's global jihadist ideology aimed to establish a pan-Islamic caliphate. The group utilized suicide bombings, hijackings, and propaganda to advance its agenda. Over the years, Al-Qaeda has morphed and splintered into various factions, posing ongoing threats worldwide.

5.2 ISIS: The Islamic State of Iraq and Syria (ISIS) emerged in the early 2010s as a radical Islamist group seeking to establish a caliphate in the Middle East. ISIS became known for its brutal tactics, including mass executions and the use of social media for recruitment and propaganda. It controlled significant territory in Iraq and Syria before facing military defeats, but it continues to inspire and coordinate attacks globally.

6.   Future Challenges and Conclusion

The relationship between non-state actors and terrorism is dynamic and continually evolving. Future challenges in countering non-state actor terrorism include the adaptation of new technologies for malicious purposes, the emergence of hybrid threats that blend terrorism with other forms of conflict, and the need for international cooperation in an increasingly interconnected world.

In conclusion, non-state actors have reshaped the landscape of global security through their involvement in terrorism. Understanding their motivations, tactics, and the challenges they pose is essential for effective counterterrorism efforts. Combating non-state actor terrorism requires a multifaceted approach that addresses the root causes of extremism, disrupts financing networks, and promotes international cooperation to prevent these actors from destabilizing regions and threatening global security.

Bioterrorism and Its Threats

The term "bioterrorism" may conjure images of a doomsday scenario, where deadly pathogens are unleashed upon unsuspecting populations, causing widespread panic and death. While such dramatic events are thankfully rare, the threat of bioterrorism remains a grave concern for governments, public health organizations, and society at large. In this comprehensive exploration, we will delve into the world of bioterrorism, examining its history, the agents involved, motivations, potential consequences, and the strategies employed to mitigate these threats.

I. Historical Context

Bioterrorism, the use of biological agents to harm or intimidate individuals, groups, or entire societies, is not a new concept. Its roots can be traced back to ancient times when besieging armies would catapult diseased animal carcasses over city walls to infect their enemies. However, modern bioterrorism is a far more sophisticated and potentially catastrophic phenomenon.

1.   Early Instances of Bioterrorism
One of the earliest recorded instances of bioterrorism dates back to the 18th century when British forces in North America attempted to spread smallpox among Native American populations by distributing infected blankets. This heinous act resulted in the deaths of thousands.
2.   The Anthrax Attacks (2001)
The most significant and widely publicized bioterrorism event in recent history occurred in the United States shortly after the 9/11 attacks. In October 2001, letters containing anthrax spores were mailed to several media outlets and two U.S. senators' offices. Five people died, and 17 others were infected. This event underscored the potential devastation that bioterrorism could cause.

II. Agents of Bioterrorism

Bioterrorists can employ a range of biological agents to achieve their malevolent goals. These agents are chosen for their ability to cause illness, death, or widespread fear. Some of the most commonly considered agents include:

1.   Anthrax (Bacillus anthracis)
Anthrax is a bacterium that can form spores, making it highly resistant to environmental factors. Inhalation of anthrax spores can lead to severe respiratory illness and death if left untreated.
2.   Smallpox (Variola virus)

Smallpox, eradicated from the natural world in 1980, exists only in laboratory stockpiles. If used as a bioweapon, it could cause a global health crisis due to a lack of immunity in the population.
3.   Botulinum Toxin (Clostridium botulinum)
Botulinum toxin is one of the most potent toxins known to humans. It can cause paralysis and death if ingested, inhaled, or absorbed through mucous membranes.
4.   Plague (Yersinia pestis)
Plague, transmitted by fleas, can cause severe respiratory symptoms when inhaled. Without treatment, it can be fatal.
5.   Ebola Virus (Ebola virus)
Ebola is a highly lethal virus that causes hemorrhagic fever. It spreads through direct contact with bodily fluids and has the potential to cause large outbreaks.

III. Motivations Behind Bioterrorism

Understanding the motivations behind bioterrorism is essential for developing effective countermeasures. Several factors drive individuals or groups to engage in bioterrorist activities:

1.   Ideological or Political Beliefs
Some bioterrorists are driven by extreme ideologies or political beliefs. They may see bioterrorism as a way to further their cause or to retaliate against perceived enemies.
2.   Religious Extremism
In some cases, religious extremist groups may employ bioterrorism as a means to achieve their goals. They may believe that such acts are sanctioned by their faith.
3.   Psychological Gratification
Bioterrorists may derive satisfaction from causing fear and harm to others. The power to inflict suffering can be a motivating factor.
4.   Revenge
Personal vendettas or a desire for revenge against a specific individual, organization, or society can motivate bioterrorists.
5.   Anonymity
Bioterrorists may believe that using biological agents allows them to remain anonymous and evade capture, making it an attractive method for those seeking to avoid accountability.

IV. Potential Consequences of Bioterrorism

The consequences of a successful bioterrorist attack can be catastrophic, impacting individuals, communities, and nations on multiple levels:

1.   Loss of Life
Bioterrorism can result in significant loss of life, especially if a highly contagious agent is used or if the targeted population lacks immunity.
2.   Public Health Crisis
The emergence of a new infectious disease due to bioterrorism can overwhelm healthcare systems, leading to a public health crisis.
3.   Economic Disruption
Bioterrorist attacks can disrupt economies by causing closures of businesses, quarantine measures, and a decline in consumer confidence.
4.   Societal Panic
The fear generated by bioterrorism can lead to societal panic, with people stockpiling supplies, avoiding public spaces, and mistrusting others.
5.   Strain on Medical Resources
Hospitals and healthcare facilities can be overwhelmed by the sudden influx of patients, leading to shortages of medical supplies and personnel.

V. Mitigating Bioterrorism Threats

Efforts to counter bioterrorism encompass a multi-faceted approach involving intelligence, public health, law enforcement, and international collaboration:

1.   Surveillance and Intelligence
Enhanced surveillance and intelligence-sharing systems help detect and prevent potential bioterrorist threats before they materialize.
2.   Strengthened Public Health Infrastructure
A robust public health system is crucial for rapid detection, response, and containment of bioterrorist incidents.
3.   Research and Development
Continued research into diagnostics, vaccines, and treatments for potential bioterror agents is essential to mitigate their impact.
4.   International Cooperation
Bioterrorism is a global threat, and international cooperation is vital for information sharing, response coordination, and the development of global norms and agreements.
5.   Preparedness and Training
First responders, healthcare workers, and law enforcement agencies should receive specialized training to effectively respond to bioterrorist incidents.
6.   Biosecurity Measures
Strict biosecurity measures in laboratories and research facilities are essential to prevent the theft or accidental release of dangerous pathogens.

Bioterrorism remains a significant threat in the modern world, and its potential consequences are grave. Vigilance, preparedness, and international cooperation are essential in mitigating these threats and ensuring the safety and security of individuals and societies. As we move forward, the continued advancement of science and technology must be accompanied by ethical considerations and responsible practices to prevent the misuse of biological agents for destructive purposes.

Case Studies and Incidents

Biological warfare, often referred to as biowarfare or bioterrorism, is a form of warfare that involves the use of biological agents to harm or kill humans, animals, or plants. This type of warfare has been employed throughout history, with varying degrees of success and impact. In this comprehensive exploration, we will delve into case studies and incidents of biological warfare, spanning from ancient times to more recent events.

The use of biological agents as weapons is not a new phenomenon. Throughout history, various civilizations and groups have sought to harness the power of pathogens and toxins to gain an advantage in conflicts. Biological warfare has evolved from crude methods involving infected corpses to sophisticated techniques that can target specific populations with deadly precision. In this examination, we will investigate notable case studies and incidents of biological warfare, shedding light on the devastating consequences and ethical dilemmas associated with this form of warfare.

Ancient Instances of Biological Warfare

1.   Siege of Caffa (1346):
The siege of Caffa, a Genoese trading colony in Crimea, is often cited as one of the earliest instances of biological warfare. During the siege, the Mongol forces outside the city reportedly catapulted the bodies of plague victims over the city walls, leading to the outbreak of the Black Death among the defenders. This tactic is said to have contributed to the spread of the pandemic in Europe.
2.   Use of Arsenic Smoke (circa 300 BC):
Ancient Chinese military texts describe the use of toxic smoke generated by burning arsenic-containing materials to poison enemy troops during sieges. This early form of chemical and biological warfare foreshadowed more advanced methods in later centuries.

Biological Warfare During the Colonial Era

3.   Blankets Infected with Smallpox (1763):
During the French and Indian War, British officers reportedly provided blankets from a smallpox hospital to Native American tribes allied with them. This deliberate act of infection aimed to weaken the indigenous population. While the extent of the success of this biological warfare tactic is debated, it highlights the unethical use of diseases as weapons.

World War I and Biological Weapons

4.   German Sabotage in the United States (1916):
Before the United States entered World War I, German agents engaged in acts of sabotage on American soil, including the release of anthrax and glanders (a disease affecting horses) in an attempt to disrupt the American war effort. These incidents underscore the global nature of early biological warfare efforts.

World War II and Japanese Biowarfare

5.   Unit 731 (1930s-1940s):
Perhaps one of the most notorious examples of biological warfare experimentation occurred in Unit 731, a covert Japanese military unit during World War II. Researchers conducted inhumane experiments on thousands of Chinese and Allied prisoners, testing biological agents like anthrax and plague. These experiments resulted in the deaths of many victims and left a dark legacy.

Cold War Era Biowarfare Programs

6.   Soviet Biopreparat (1970s-1990s):
The Soviet Union operated a vast and secretive bioweapons program known as Biopreparat during the Cold War. This program aimed to develop deadly pathogens, including smallpox, anthrax, and Marburg virus, for potential use in warfare. The existence of this program was revealed in the 1990s, leading to international condemnation and disarmament efforts.

Contemporary Concerns and Incidents

7.   Amerithrax Attacks (2001):
In the wake of the 9/11 terrorist attacks, the United States experienced a series of anthrax-laden letters mailed to various individuals and organizations. This bioterrorism incident, known as the Amerithrax attacks, killed five people and raised concerns about the accessibility of biological agents to malicious actors.
8.   Syrian Civil War and Chemical Weapons (2010s):
While not strictly biological warfare, the Syrian civil war witnessed the use of chemical agents, including sarin gas and chlorine, against civilian populations. These attacks, attributed to the Syrian government, raised international outrage and highlighted the blurred lines between chemical and biological warfare.

Contemporary Bioweapons Threats

9.   Emerging Infectious Diseases and Bioweapons Potential:
In recent years, the world has grappled with the threat of naturally occurring infectious diseases like Ebola, Zika, and COVID-19. These outbreaks have underscored the potential for pathogens to spread globally and have raised concerns about their deliberate misuse as bioweapons.

The Ethics and Challenges of Biological Warfare

The use of biological warfare raises profound ethical questions. It blurs the line between conventional warfare and acts of terrorism. Some of the key ethical dilemmas include:

•   Indiscriminate Nature: Biological agents often do not discriminate between combatants and civilians, making their use inherently unethical.
•   Lack of Control: Once released, biological agents can be challenging to control, potentially causing unintended harm to the perpetrators or their allies.
•   Global Consequences: Biological warfare can have global repercussions, with the potential to trigger pandemics that affect populations far beyond the intended targets.
•   Legitimacy and Accountability: Determining who is responsible for bioweapon attacks can be difficult, leading to challenges in assigning blame and seeking justice.

International Efforts to Prevent Biological Warfare

The international community has taken steps to prevent the use of biological weapons:

•   Biological Weapons Convention (BWC): Adopted in 1972, the BWC prohibits the development, production, and stockpiling of biological weapons and their delivery systems. While it lacks robust verification mechanisms, it serves as a foundational treaty.
•   The Australia Group: This informal forum of countries aims to control the export of materials and technologies that could be used to develop biological or chemical weapons.
•   UN Security Council Resolutions: The United Nations Security Council has passed resolutions condemning the use of chemical and biological weapons and imposing sanctions on violators.

Biological warfare, with its long and dark history, remains a persistent threat to global security and ethics. While international efforts have sought to curtail the development and use of biological weapons, the evolving nature of science and technology presents ongoing challenges in maintaining effective controls. The case studies and incidents presented here underscore the need for continued vigilance, diplomacy, and ethical consideration in the realm of biological warfare. Only through collective action can we hope to prevent the devastating consequences of this form of warfare in the future.

The Science of Epidemics and Pandemics

Epidemics and pandemics have shaped the course of human history for centuries. From the Black Death in the 14th century to the COVID-19 pandemic in the 21st century, infectious diseases have had profound effects on societies, economies, and public health. Understanding the science behind epidemics and pandemics is crucial not only for responding effectively but also for preventing and mitigating their impact. In this comprehensive exploration, we will delve into the science of epidemics and pandemics, examining the causes, dynamics, and responses to these global health crises.

Section 1: What Are Epidemics and Pandemics?

Epidemics and pandemics are not just medical terms; they are complex events with distinct definitions.

An epidemic refers to the sudden increase in the number of cases of a particular disease within a population. It's a localized outbreak that can occur in a single community or region.

A pandemic, on the other hand, is a global outbreak of a disease, typically caused by a novel pathogen to which most people have little or no immunity. Pandemics are marked by widespread transmission, affecting multiple countries and continents.

Section 2: The Role of Pathogens

Understanding the science of epidemics and pandemics begins with an examination of the pathogens responsible for these events. Pathogens can be bacteria, viruses, fungi, or parasites. They have distinct properties that determine how they spread and the diseases they cause.

Section 3: Transmission Dynamics

The spread of infectious diseases is governed by complex transmission dynamics. Factors such as the reproductive number (R0), incubation period, and modes of transmission play critical roles in determining the speed and extent of an outbreak.

Section 4: Host-Pathogen Interactions

The susceptibility of individuals to infection varies based on their immune systems, genetics, and other factors. Understanding these host-pathogen interactions is crucial for predicting how a disease will impact different populations.

Section 5: Historical Epidemics and Pandemics

To appreciate the science behind epidemics and pandemics, it's essential to examine historical examples. We'll explore how events like the Spanish flu, HIV/AIDS, and the bubonic plague have shaped our understanding of infectious diseases.

Section 6: Modern Pandemics

The 21st century has witnessed several significant pandemics, including the H1N1 influenza pandemic in 2009 and the COVID-19 pandemic that began in 2019. These events have highlighted the global interconnectedness of our world and the challenges of responding to novel pathogens.

Section 7: Epidemiology and Disease Surveillance

Epidemiologists play a crucial role in tracking and controlling epidemics and pandemics. They use mathematical models, data analysis, and field investigations to understand how diseases spread and to inform public health responses.

Section 8: Vaccination and Immunization

Vaccination is one of the most effective tools for preventing epidemics and pandemics. We'll explore the science of vaccines, including how they work, the development process, and the challenges of achieving widespread vaccination coverage.

Section 9: Antimicrobial Resistance

The misuse and overuse of antibiotics have led to the rise of antimicrobial resistance (AMR), which poses a significant threat to our ability to treat infectious diseases. Understanding AMR and finding solutions is a critical aspect of epidemic and pandemic science.

Section 10: Pandemic Preparedness and Response

Preventing and mitigating the impact of pandemics requires preparedness and swift response. We'll delve into the strategies and technologies used to contain outbreaks and protect public health.

Section 11: Socioeconomic and Ethical Implications

Epidemics and pandemics have far-reaching societal and ethical implications. We'll examine issues such as healthcare access, misinformation, and the balance between public health measures and individual rights.

Section 12: The Future of Epidemics and Pandemics

Finally, we'll discuss what the future might hold in terms of epidemic and pandemic science. How will climate change, globalization, and advances in healthcare technology impact the dynamics of infectious diseases?

The science of epidemics and pandemics is a multidisciplinary field that draws on biology, epidemiology, sociology, and more. It's a dynamic and ever-evolving area of study that continues to be of utmost importance in our interconnected world. By understanding the causes and mechanisms of these global health crises, we can better prepare for and respond to the inevitable epidemics and pandemics of the future.

Anatomy of an Epidemic

In the modern world, epidemics have become an ominous part of our collective consciousness. These widespread outbreaks of diseases or health crises can be devastating, affecting millions of lives and often challenging the very foundations of our healthcare systems. The term "epidemic" conjures images of infectious diseases sweeping through communities, but in today's context, it encompasses a broader range of health challenges, including mental health disorders, chronic illnesses, and addiction.

To understand the anatomy of an epidemic, we must delve deep into its multifaceted nature. Epidemics are not isolated events but rather complex phenomena influenced by a confluence of factors—biological, environmental, societal, and even economic. This exploration will take us on a journey through history, examining epidemics of the past, and into the present, where new types of epidemics have emerged. We'll analyze the roles of science, healthcare systems, public policy, and societal attitudes in shaping and responding to epidemics.

I. Historical Epidemics

A. Infectious Disease Epidemics

1.   The Black Death: A Lesson from History
•   The devastating impact of the bubonic plague in the 14th century.
•   Factors contributing to the rapid spread of the disease.
•   Socioeconomic consequences and changes in healthcare practices.
2.   The Spanish Flu of 1918: A Modern Pandemic
•   The emergence and global spread of the H1N1 influenza virus.
•   The social and economic repercussions of the Spanish flu.
•   Lessons learned and their implications for future pandemics.

B. Mental Health Epidemics

1.   The Shell-Shock Epidemic: World War I and Psychological Trauma
•   The emergence of shell shock as a widespread psychological disorder.
•   The societal response and evolving understanding of trauma.
•   Parallels with contemporary mental health issues among veterans.
2.   The Opioid Epidemic: A Modern Tragedy
•   The roots and evolution of the opioid epidemic in the United States.
•   The role of pharmaceutical companies, healthcare providers, and patients.

- Efforts to combat the epidemic and their effectiveness.

II. Modern Epidemics

A. Chronic Illness Epidemics

1. The Diabetes Epidemic: Uncontrolled Metabolism
- The rising prevalence of diabetes worldwide.
- Contributing factors, including lifestyle and genetics.
- The economic and healthcare burdens associated with diabetes.
2. Obesity Epidemic: A Weighty Issue
- The global increase in obesity rates.
- The complex interplay of genetics, environment, and behavior.
- Strategies for prevention and intervention.

B. Mental Health Epidemics

1. The Anxiety Epidemic: Navigating Modern Stresses
- The surge in anxiety disorders and their impact on individuals and society.
- Examinations of societal factors, including social media and economic stress.
- Approaches to destigmatizing mental health and improving access to care.
2. The Alzheimer's Epidemic: Unraveling the Mind
- The aging population and the prevalence of Alzheimer's disease.
- Advances in research and potential treatments.
- The ethical and societal implications of Alzheimer's care.

III. Anatomy of an Epidemic: Contributing Factors

A. The Role of Science and Research

1. Epidemiology and Modeling: Predicting and Understanding Epidemics
- The science of tracking and predicting disease outbreaks.
- The importance of data collection, analysis, and modeling.
- The role of modern technology in enhancing epidemiological research.
2. Advances in Medicine: From Vaccines to Treatments
- The historical and contemporary significance of vaccines.
- Breakthroughs in treatment and their impact on epidemic control.
- Challenges in equitable access to medical advancements.

B. Healthcare Systems and Infrastructure

1.   Healthcare Access and Disparities
- The relationship between healthcare access and epidemic control.
- Disparities in healthcare provision and their effects on vulnerable populations.
- Strategies to address healthcare inequalities.
    2.   Hospital Preparedness and Surge Capacity
- The challenges faced by healthcare facilities during epidemics.
- The importance of surge capacity planning and pandemic preparedness.
- Lessons from recent epidemics, including COVID-19.

C. Public Policy and Governance

1.   Government Response and Crisis Management
- The role of governments in addressing epidemics.
- The balance between individual rights and public health measures.
- Case studies of effective and ineffective government responses.

2.   International Collaboration and Pandemic Diplomacy
- The importance of global cooperation in epidemic control.
- The role of international organizations like the WHO.
- Challenges in achieving consensus and equitable distribution of resources.

IV. Social Attitudes and Stigma

A. Stigmatization of Epidemics

1.   Social Stigma and Infectious Diseases
- The history of stigma associated with diseases like HIV/AIDS.
- The impact of stigma on prevention, testing, and treatment.
- Efforts to combat disease-related stigma.

2.   Mental Health Stigma: Silence and Suffering
- The pervasive stigma surrounding mental health issues.
- The consequences of stigma on individuals seeking help.
- Initiatives to reduce mental health stigma and promote awareness.

B. Communication and Media

1.   Information Spread and Misinformation
- The role of media in shaping public perceptions of epidemics.
- The spread of misinformation and conspiracy theories.
- Strategies for responsible journalism during epidemics.

2.   Fear, Panic, and Public Behavior
- The psychological impact of media coverage on public behavior.

- The challenge of balancing information and fear management.
- Lessons from past epidemics for media and public communication.

V. Conclusion: Lessons Learned and Future Directions

A. The Need for Interdisciplinary Approaches

1. Collaborative Research and Data Sharing
- The importance of breaking down silos between scientific disciplines.
- Encouraging collaboration between epidemiologists, clinicians, social scientists, and policymakers.
- Promoting data sharing and open science.

B. Building Resilient Healthcare Systems

1. Strengthening Healthcare Infrastructure
- Investments in healthcare infrastructure and workforce.
- Preparing for future epidemics and disasters.
- Addressing the root causes of chronic illnesses and mental health challenges.

C. Shaping Societal Attitudes

1. Promoting Empathy and Understanding
- Fostering empathy and reducing stigma in society.
- Supporting individuals and communities affected by epidemics.
- Elevating the importance of mental health and holistic well-being.

D. The Role of Global Cooperation

1. Strengthening International Collaboration
- Reevaluating international governance structures.
- Ensuring equitable access to vaccines and treatments.
- Addressing global health disparities and climate change as drivers of epidemics.

In this comprehensive exploration of the anatomy of an epidemic, we've journeyed through history, analyzing the complexities of past and present health crises. Epidemics are not isolated events but reflections of the interconnectedness of our world. They demand interdisciplinary solutions, resilience in healthcare systems, compassionate social attitudes, and international cooperation. The lessons learned from these epidemics should guide our path forward, as we strive to prevent and respond to the health challenges of the future.

The task of addressing epidemics is ongoing, and the knowledge gained from each crisis should serve as a beacon, guiding us toward a healthier, more resilient, and equitable future. As we conclude this exploration of the anatomy of an epidemic, let's reflect on some key takeaways and the directions we should pursue in the years to come.

I. Acknowledging Complexity

Epidemics are intricate phenomena that rarely have a single cause or solution. They manifest across a spectrum, from infectious diseases to chronic illnesses and mental health disorders. This complexity necessitates a holistic understanding that encompasses biological, environmental, societal, and economic factors. To effectively combat epidemics, we must acknowledge and address this complexity.

II. The Power of Science and Research

Scientific research has played a pivotal role in our ability to understand, predict, and mitigate epidemics. Advances in epidemiology, virology, and medical treatments have saved countless lives. To continue this progress, we must continue to invest in research, data collection, and technological innovations. Moreover, interdisciplinary collaboration between scientists, healthcare professionals, and social scientists is essential to unravel the complexities of epidemics fully.

III. Strengthening Healthcare Systems

The COVID-19 pandemic laid bare the vulnerabilities in healthcare systems worldwide. Inadequate infrastructure, shortages of medical supplies, and overburdened healthcare workers hindered our response. Building resilient healthcare systems means investing in infrastructure, expanding healthcare access, and prioritizing the well-being of healthcare workers. Preparedness for future epidemics, both in terms of surge capacity and supply chain resilience, is paramount.

IV. Addressing Social Stigma

Stigma surrounding epidemics can be as damaging as the diseases themselves. It can deter individuals from seeking care, hinder prevention efforts, and exacerbate mental health challenges. To address this, we must actively work to reduce stigma through public education campaigns, open conversations, and empathetic support for affected individuals. Shifting societal attitudes toward understanding and compassion is an essential component of epidemic control.

V. Global Cooperation

In our interconnected world, epidemics know no borders. They demand international cooperation and solidarity. Global health organizations, such as the World Health Organization (WHO), play a pivotal role in coordinating responses and ensuring equitable access to resources. However, international collaboration must go beyond healthcare; it should encompass broader challenges like climate change and social determinants of health that can drive epidemics.

VI. Prevention and Preparedness

While effective responses to epidemics are crucial, we should place greater emphasis on prevention and preparedness. This includes strategies to reduce the risk of epidemics, such as vaccination programs and lifestyle interventions. It also means developing robust pandemic preparedness plans that can be swiftly activated when needed.

VII. Mental Health and Well-Being

Mental health is an integral part of overall well-being, and epidemics often take a toll on mental health. Our understanding of mental health issues has evolved, and we must continue to destigmatize these conditions and ensure that mental health services are accessible to all. Moreover, recognizing the psychological impact of epidemics on individuals and communities is essential for comprehensive care.

VIII. Building Resilience

Building resilience is not just about responding to epidemics but also about addressing the underlying vulnerabilities in our societies. This includes reducing health disparities, addressing social determinants of health, and mitigating the impacts of climate change. Resilience is a long-term endeavor that requires sustained commitment.

In conclusion, the anatomy of an epidemic is a complex interplay of factors that challenges our society's ability to respond effectively. Epidemics of the past and present have taught us valuable lessons about the importance of science, healthcare infrastructure, societal attitudes, and global cooperation. As we navigate the future, these lessons must guide our actions.

The task of addressing epidemics is ongoing, and it requires a united effort from individuals, communities, governments, and the global community. By acknowledging the complexity of epidemics, investing in research and healthcare systems, combating stigma, fostering global cooperation, emphasizing prevention and resilience, and prioritizing mental health, we can collectively work towards a world where epidemics are less frequent, less severe, and better managed. It is a challenging journey, but it is one that we must undertake for the sake of the health and well-being of present and future generations.

Factors Leading to Epidemics

Epidemics, characterized by the rapid and widespread outbreak of infectious diseases, have plagued humanity throughout history. These events have often resulted in devastating consequences, both in terms of human lives lost and economic and social disruptions. Understanding the factors leading to epidemics is crucial for preventing and mitigating their impact. In this comprehensive exploration, we will delve into the multifaceted elements that contribute to the emergence and propagation of epidemics.

Introduction

Epidemics, whether caused by familiar pathogens like influenza or newly emerging threats like the novel coronavirus (SARS-CoV-2), have been a recurrent feature of human history. These events have shaped societies, altered the course of wars, and influenced the rise and fall of civilizations. The factors that lead to epidemics are complex and interconnected, often encompassing biological, environmental, social, and political dimensions. To understand these factors, we must examine them individually and appreciate their interplay.

Biological Factors

1.   Pathogen Characteristics: The nature of the pathogen itself plays a pivotal role in the emergence of epidemics. Pathogens with high transmission rates, such as the measles virus, can quickly infect a large number of individuals. Meanwhile, pathogens that mutate rapidly, like the influenza virus, can escape immune responses and develop resistance to treatment.
2.   Zoonotic Transmission: Many epidemics originate from zoonotic transmission, where pathogens jump from animals to humans. Factors like increased human-animal interactions, deforestation, and the wildlife trade can facilitate this transmission. For instance, the HIV/AIDS pandemic likely emerged from the hunting and consumption of infected primates.
3.   Antibiotic Resistance: The misuse and overuse of antibiotics have led to the development of antibiotic-resistant pathogens, making infections harder to treat. Epidemics caused by drug-resistant bacteria, such as methicillin-resistant Staphylococcus aureus (MRSA), are a growing concern.

Environmental Factors

4.   Climate Change: Altered climate patterns can affect the distribution and behavior of disease vectors (e.g., mosquitoes carrying malaria). Rising temperatures and

changing rainfall patterns can expand the geographic range of vector-borne diseases, contributing to epidemics in previously unaffected areas.

5.	Urbanization: Rapid urbanization can lead to overcrowding, inadequate sanitation, and poor living conditions, creating ideal environments for disease transmission. Megacities around the world often struggle to control epidemics due to these factors.

Social Factors

6.	Globalization: The ease of travel and trade in the modern world allows pathogens to spread quickly across borders. An infected individual in one part of the world can lead to an epidemic in another within a matter of hours or days.

7.	Healthcare Infrastructure: The quality and accessibility of healthcare services can significantly impact the course of an epidemic. Regions with limited healthcare infrastructure may struggle to diagnose, treat, and contain diseases effectively, leading to larger outbreaks.

8.	Vaccine Hesitancy: Mistrust in vaccines and low vaccine coverage rates can facilitate the resurgence of vaccine-preventable diseases. Outbreaks of diseases like measles have occurred in areas with low vaccination rates.

Political and Economic Factors

9.	Political Stability: Political instability and conflict can disrupt healthcare systems and hinder epidemic response efforts. Regions affected by war or civil unrest may struggle to control disease outbreaks.

10.	Economic Disparities: Socioeconomic disparities can influence an individual's access to healthcare and ability to follow preventive measures. Vulnerable populations often bear the brunt of epidemics, as seen with COVID-19's disproportionate impact on marginalized communities.

11.	Global Health Policy: International cooperation and adherence to global health policies are critical in preventing epidemics. Failures in coordination, as witnessed during the early stages of the COVID-19 pandemic, can allow diseases to spread unchecked.

Human Behavior

12.	Hygiene Practices: Personal hygiene, such as handwashing and sanitation, is essential in preventing the spread of infectious diseases. Poor hygiene practices can contribute to the rapid transmission of pathogens.

13.   Travel Behavior: The movement of people, whether for leisure or work, can introduce pathogens to new regions. Travel restrictions and quarantine measures have been used to mitigate this risk during epidemics.

14.   Social Distancing: During outbreaks, social distancing measures can slow the spread of disease. Compliance with these measures can vary widely based on cultural norms and government policies.

Technology and Communication

15.   Advancements in Diagnostics: Access to rapid diagnostic tools can aid in early detection and containment of epidemics. Technologies like PCR testing and gene sequencing have been instrumental in identifying and characterizing novel pathogens.

16.   Information Dissemination: The internet and social media can spread information about epidemics rapidly. While this can help raise awareness and encourage preventive measures, it can also lead to the rapid spread of misinformation and panic.

Epidemics are the result of a complex interplay of biological, environmental, social, political, economic, and behavioral factors. While it is impossible to eliminate all risks, a comprehensive understanding of these factors is essential for epidemic preparedness and response.

Efforts to prevent and control epidemics must be multidisciplinary, involving cooperation between governments, healthcare systems, scientists, and the public. Investment in healthcare infrastructure, research, and international collaboration is crucial in mitigating the impact of epidemics on human health and society as a whole.

The lessons learned from past epidemics, including the ongoing COVID-19 pandemic, highlight the need for continuous vigilance and preparedness in the face of emerging infectious diseases. Only through a concerted global effort can we hope to reduce the frequency and severity of epidemics in the future.

Outbreak Investigation

Outbreaks of infectious diseases have shaped the course of human history, with pandemics and epidemics leaving indelible marks on societies and economies. From the Black Death in the 14th century to the 1918 influenza pandemic and more recently, the COVID-19 pandemic, these events have underscored the need for robust outbreak investigation and management. This comprehensive exploration delves into the fundamental aspects of outbreak investigations during pandemics and epidemics, examining their significance, key stages, methods, challenges, and the vital role of public health interventions.

I. Understanding Pandemics and Epidemics

To initiate our discussion, we must first establish a clear understanding of what constitutes a pandemic and an epidemic.

1.   Pandemic:
A pandemic is a global outbreak of a disease, typically caused by a novel pathogen to which a large portion of the population has little or no immunity. These events affect multiple countries and regions, causing widespread illness and often severe socio-economic disruptions.
2.   Epidemic:
An epidemic, on the other hand, is the occurrence of cases of a disease in a population that is greater than what is normally expected. While epidemics can be localized, they may also affect large areas or entire countries.

II. The Significance of Outbreak Investigation

Outbreak investigation is crucial for several reasons:

1.   Early Detection and Response:
Rapid identification of outbreaks is essential to implement timely interventions, preventing further transmission and minimizing the impact on public health.
2.   Understanding Transmission Dynamics:
Investigating outbreaks provides insights into how diseases spread, including routes of transmission, susceptible populations, and the role of asymptomatic carriers.
3.   Resource Allocation:
Effective allocation of resources, such as medical supplies, personnel, and healthcare facilities, is dependent on accurate outbreak investigation data.
4.   Policy Development:

Data from outbreak investigations inform the development of public health policies, including vaccination campaigns and quarantine measures.

5.   Public Awareness:

Transparent and accurate reporting during outbreaks helps to manage public perception and reduce panic or misinformation.

III. Key Stages of Outbreak Investigation

Successful outbreak investigations follow a series of critical stages:

1.   Initial Detection:

The process begins with the recognition of an unusual cluster of cases or a sudden increase in disease incidence. Health systems, surveillance, and vigilant healthcare workers play a pivotal role in this phase.

2.   Verification:

Health authorities must confirm that an outbreak is indeed occurring and determine the causative agent. Laboratory testing and case definition development are key components.

3.   Epidemiological Studies:

Field investigations involve epidemiologists gathering data about affected individuals, including demographics, travel history, contacts, and symptoms. This information helps identify the source of the outbreak and the mode of transmission.

4.   Hypothesis Generation:

Based on the data collected, hypotheses are developed regarding the source of the outbreak. These hypotheses guide subsequent investigations.

5.   Testing Hypotheses:

Further studies, including case-control studies and environmental assessments, are conducted to test hypotheses. These studies provide evidence to support or refute potential sources and transmission routes.

6.   Control Measures:

Once the source and mode of transmission are identified, control measures are implemented. These may include isolation of cases, quarantine of contacts, vaccination campaigns, or public health messaging.

7.   Data Analysis and Reporting:

All data collected are analyzed to refine the understanding of the outbreak. Regular updates and transparent reporting are essential for effective communication with the public and stakeholders.

IV. Methods and Tools in Outbreak Investigation

Several methods and tools are employed during outbreak investigations:

1.   Epidemiological Surveys:
These surveys involve collecting data from affected individuals and their contacts to determine patterns and risk factors.
2.   Laboratory Testing:
Molecular biology techniques, such as PCR, are used to identify the causative agent. Serological testing can reveal immunity levels in the population.
3.   Geographic Information Systems (GIS):
GIS is used to map cases geographically, helping identify hotspots and potential sources of infection.
4.   Genomic Sequencing:
In modern outbreak investigations, genomic sequencing of pathogens can pinpoint the source and track transmission chains.
5.   Simulation Models:
Mathematical models help predict disease spread and assess the impact of interventions.

V. Challenges in Outbreak Investigation

Outbreak investigations are not without challenges:

1.   Data Quality:
Timely and accurate data collection can be hindered by limited resources, infrastructure, or political factors.
2.   Cross-Border Coordination:
Pandemics often transcend borders, necessitating international cooperation, which can be complex and politically sensitive.
3.   Public Compliance:
Implementing control measures relies on public compliance, which can be challenging, especially in the face of misinformation.
4.   Resource Constraints:
Outbreak investigations demand substantial resources, including skilled personnel, laboratory facilities, and funding.
5.   Ethical Dilemmas:
Balancing public health measures with individual rights and privacy can pose ethical dilemmas.

VI. Public Health Interventions

Outbreak investigations inform the design and implementation of public health interventions:

1.   Isolation and Quarantine:
Infected individuals are isolated, and their contacts are quarantined to limit transmission.
2.   Vaccination Campaigns:
Immunization can be a crucial tool in preventing outbreaks, especially for vaccine-preventable diseases.
3.   Health Education:
Public awareness campaigns provide information on disease prevention and control measures.
4.   Travel Restrictions:
In some cases, travel restrictions may be imposed to prevent the spread of disease across borders.
5.   Antiviral Medications:
Medications can be administered to treat infected individuals and reduce transmission.
6.   Environmental Control:
Sanitary measures, such as water treatment and vector control, can be implemented to prevent disease transmission.

VII. Case Studies: Learning from the Past

To illustrate the importance of outbreak investigation, let's examine two significant historical outbreaks:

1.   The 1918 Influenza Pandemic:
The 1918 influenza pandemic, often referred to as the Spanish flu, infected one-third of the world's population and resulted in millions of deaths. Outbreak investigations were limited at the time due to limited scientific knowledge and communication. However, modern analysis of preserved samples revealed that the virus likely originated in birds and mutated to infect humans. This knowledge informs current pandemic preparedness.
2.   The COVID-19 Pandemic:
The COVID-19 pandemic, caused by the novel coronavirus SARS-CoV-2, is a contemporary example. Rigorous outbreak investigations were conducted worldwide to identify the source of the virus, understand its transmission dynamics, and develop effective control measures. Genomic sequencing played a pivotal role in tracking the virus's evolution and spread.

VIII. Lessons for the Future

Outbreak investigations provide invaluable lessons for the future:

1.   Invest in Surveillance Systems:
Strengthening disease surveillance systems and early warning mechanisms is critical for rapid outbreak detection.

2.   Global Collaboration:
International cooperation and information sharing are essential to combat pandemics effectively.

3.   Invest in Research and Technology:
Advances in genomics, modeling, and laboratory techniques enhance our ability to investigate and respond to outbreaks.

4.   Public Health Education:
Public health authorities should invest in educating the public about disease prevention, the importance of vaccinations, and how to respond to outbreaks responsibly.

5.   Adaptive Preparedness:
Preparedness plans should be adaptable and flexible to respond to different types of outbreaks, from novel pathogens to resurgences of known diseases.

6.   Ethical Frameworks:
Developing clear ethical frameworks for outbreak response can guide decision-making in times of crisis, ensuring that individual rights are respected while protecting public health.

7.   Investment in Healthcare Infrastructure:
Strengthening healthcare infrastructure, including laboratory capacities and healthcare facilities, is crucial to respond effectively to outbreaks.

8.   Risk Communication:
Effective risk communication strategies should be developed and practiced to ensure that the public receives accurate information during outbreaks, reducing panic and misinformation.

9.   Community Engagement:
Engaging communities in outbreak response efforts fosters cooperation and compliance with control measures.

Outbreak investigation is a multifaceted process that plays a central role in mitigating the impact of pandemics and epidemics. From understanding the basics of what constitutes a pandemic and an epidemic to recognizing the significance of outbreak investigation, the key stages involved, the methods and tools utilized, the challenges faced, and the importance of public health interventions, this exploration underscores the critical role that public health officials, epidemiologists, and healthcare workers play in safeguarding global health.

History has shown that outbreaks of infectious diseases are not only inevitable but also have the potential to be devastating. By learning from the past and adapting to new challenges, we can better prepare for future outbreaks. Timely and effective outbreak investigations, informed by science, data, and cooperation, are essential in our ongoing battle against pandemics and epidemics. In an interconnected world, the health of one nation is inextricably linked to the health of all, making robust outbreak investigations a cornerstone of global health security.

The Global Challenge of Pandemics

Pandemics are a recurring challenge that has haunted humanity throughout history. These global health crises not only claim lives but also disrupt societies and economies. The COVID-19 pandemic of 2019-2021 is a stark reminder of the devastating impact pandemics can have on the world. This essay explores the global challenge of pandemics, examining their causes, consequences, and the strategies employed to combat them.

I. The Historical Context

Pandemics are not a modern phenomenon. They have been a part of human history for centuries. One of the earliest recorded pandemics was the Antonine Plague in the 2nd century AD, which is believed to have been smallpox or measles. The Black Death of the 14th century, caused by the bacterium Yersinia pestis, wiped out an estimated 75-200 million people in Eurasia. These historical pandemics shaped societies, altered the course of wars, and left indelible marks on culture and art.

II. Causes of Pandemics

A. Zoonotic Origins

Many pandemics have their origins in animals, a phenomenon known as zoonotic spillover. Diseases like HIV, Ebola, and COVID-19 are believed to have originated in animals before jumping to humans. Factors such as deforestation, urbanization, and wildlife trade increase the likelihood of these spillover events. Encroachment into natural habitats brings humans into closer contact with animals, facilitating the transmission of pathogens.

B. Globalization

The interconnectedness of the modern world through trade and travel accelerates the spread of infectious diseases. A person infected with a virus in one corner of the globe can travel to the opposite side within hours, carrying the pathogen with them. This globalization effect has made containment and mitigation of pandemics more challenging.

C. Antibiotic Resistance

The overuse and misuse of antibiotics have led to the emergence of drug-resistant bacteria. Antibiotic-resistant infections can become pandemic if left unchecked. Diseases that were once easily treatable, like tuberculosis, are regaining their deadly status due to antibiotic resistance.

III. Consequences of Pandemics

A. Human Toll

Pandemics inflict a heavy human toll, causing illness and death on a massive scale. Families and communities are torn apart as loved ones succumb to disease. COVID-19 alone has claimed millions of lives and left countless survivors with long-lasting health complications.

B. Economic Disruption

Pandemics disrupt economies on a global scale. Lockdowns, travel restrictions, and decreased consumer confidence lead to job losses and business closures. The economic fallout from pandemics can last for years, affecting industries from tourism to manufacturing.

C. Strain on Healthcare Systems

Healthcare systems strain under the pressure of a pandemic. Hospitals become overwhelmed, facing shortages of beds, ventilators, and medical personnel. Non-COVID healthcare services also suffer as resources are diverted to pandemic response.

D. Social and Psychological Impact

Pandemics have a profound impact on mental health. Fear, anxiety, and social isolation become prevalent. The loss of routine and social interactions takes a toll on individuals and communities, leading to increased mental health issues.

E. Educational Disruption

Pandemics disrupt education, with school closures affecting millions of students. The digital divide exacerbates inequalities in access to remote learning. The long-term consequences of interrupted education can be severe.

IV. Strategies to Combat Pandemics

A. Early Detection and Surveillance

Timely detection of outbreaks is crucial. Advances in technology, such as machine learning and genetic sequencing, have improved our ability to monitor and identify novel pathogens quickly. Surveillance systems like the Global Public Health Intelligence Network (GPHIN) play a vital role in this.

B. Vaccination

Vaccination is one of the most effective tools against pandemics. The development and distribution of vaccines, as seen in the case of COVID-19, can help build herd immunity and curb the spread of the virus. However, challenges like vaccine hesitancy and equitable distribution must be addressed.

C. Antiviral Drugs

Antiviral drugs can treat and mitigate the effects of pandemics. Research into broad-spectrum antiviral drugs that can target a range of viruses is ongoing. These drugs can be vital in managing outbreaks until vaccines are widely available.

D. International Cooperation

Pandemics are global problems that require international cooperation. Organizations like the World Health Organization (WHO) and initiatives like COVAX aim to promote global collaboration in pandemic response. Sharing information, resources, and expertise across borders is essential.

E. Public Health Measures

Non-pharmaceutical interventions, such as mask-wearing, social distancing, and hand hygiene, play a critical role in slowing the spread of a virus. Public health campaigns are vital in promoting these measures and encouraging compliance.

F. Preparedness and Research

Investment in pandemic preparedness and research is essential. This includes developing rapid diagnostic tests, improving the production and distribution of personal protective equipment (PPE), and conducting research on potential pandemic pathogens.

V. Challenges and Future Outlook

A. Vaccine Equity

Ensuring equitable access to vaccines remains a major challenge. Disparities in vaccine distribution between wealthy and low-income countries highlight the need for global solidarity in addressing pandemics.

B. Misinformation

Misinformation and conspiracy theories can undermine pandemic response efforts. Promoting science-based information and combating falsehoods is a continuous battle.

C. Future Pandemic Threats

As long as zoonotic spillover events and other factors persist, pandemics will remain a threat. Vigilance, preparedness, and a commitment to learning from past pandemics are essential to mitigate future risks.

D. Climate Change

Climate change can influence the emergence and spread of infectious diseases. Rising temperatures can expand the geographic range of disease vectors like mosquitoes, leading to the spread of diseases like malaria and dengue.

The global challenge of pandemics is a complex and ongoing threat to humanity. History has shown that pandemics can shape the course of civilizations and alter the trajectory of societies. While the world has made significant progress in understanding and combating infectious diseases, the COVID-19 pandemic serves as a stark reminder of our vulnerability. Addressing the causes, consequences, and strategies to combat pandemics requires global cooperation, innovation, and a commitment to safeguarding the health and well-being of all people. The lessons learned from past pandemics must guide our actions in the face of future challenges.

Pandemics Throughout History

Pandemics are a recurring theme in human history. From the plague of Athens in 430 BCE to the COVID-19 pandemic in the 21st century, infectious diseases have shaped societies, altered the course of wars, and challenged our understanding of science and medicine. In this extensive exploration, we will journey through the annals of history, examining the most significant pandemics, their causes, consequences, and the lessons they have left behind.

1.   The Antonine Plague (165-180 CE)

The Antonine Plague, also known as the Plague of Galen, struck the Roman Empire during the reign of Emperor Marcus Aurelius. It's believed to have been either smallpox or measles, and it devastated the empire, killing millions. This pandemic had far-reaching consequences, including economic disruption, depopulation, and social unrest. The weakened Roman military contributed to their struggles against invading barbarian tribes, contributing to the eventual fall of the Western Roman Empire.

2.   The Justinian Plague (541-542 CE)

Named after the Byzantine Emperor Justinian I, this pandemic was caused by the Yersinia pestis bacterium, responsible for the bubonic plague. It swept through the Eastern Roman Empire (Byzantine Empire), killing an estimated 25-50 million people, including the Emperor himself. The economic and societal impact was profound, leading to labor shortages and the weakening of the empire. This plague left a lasting imprint on history, influencing art, literature, and religious beliefs.

3.   The Black Death (1347-1351 CE)

The Black Death, another outbreak of the bubonic plague, is one of the most infamous pandemics in history. Originating in Asia, it swept through Europe, Asia, and Africa, wiping out an estimated 75-200 million people, or 30-60% of Europe's population. This pandemic led to significant social, economic, and religious changes. Labor shortages gave peasants more bargaining power, contributing to the end of feudalism. It also spurred scientific inquiry and new medical practices.

4.   The Third Cholera Pandemic (1852-1860)

Cholera, a waterborne disease, caused multiple pandemics throughout the 19th century. The Third Cholera Pandemic, originating in India, spread globally. John Snow, a British physician, made pioneering contributions during this pandemic by tracing the source of the outbreak to contaminated water in London. His work laid the foundation for modern epidemiology and the understanding of disease transmission.

5.   The Spanish Flu (1918-1919)

The Spanish flu, caused by an H1N1 influenza A virus, remains one of the deadliest pandemics in history. It infected approximately one-third of the global population and resulted in an estimated 50 million deaths worldwide. Despite its name, the origins of the virus remain unclear. This pandemic had a profound impact on public health policies, leading to advancements in vaccine development and the establishment of the World Health Organization (WHO) in 1948.

6.   HIV/AIDS Pandemic (1980s-Present)

The HIV/AIDS pandemic began in the late 20th century and continues to affect millions of people worldwide. The virus, which attacks the immune system, has claimed over 36 million lives since the start of the epidemic. HIV/AIDS has not only challenged the medical and scientific communities but also sparked social and political controversies. It led to significant advancements in antiretroviral therapy and raised awareness about the importance of safe sex and public health measures.

7.   COVID-19 Pandemic (2019-Present)

The COVID-19 pandemic, caused by the novel coronavirus SARS-CoV-2, has reshaped the world in ways still unfolding as of my last knowledge update in September 2021. Originating in Wuhan, China, this pandemic has infected millions and caused significant loss of life. It has strained healthcare systems, triggered economic crises, and sparked debates on public health policies, vaccine distribution, and global cooperation. The pandemic's long-term impact on society, economics, and healthcare remains a subject of ongoing study.

8.   Lessons Learned

Throughout history, pandemics have exposed vulnerabilities in societies and driven innovation in science and medicine. Here are some key lessons learned from these historical pandemics:

•   Preparedness: Early detection, rapid response, and global collaboration are critical in containing pandemics.

•   Public Health: Strong public health systems, including vaccination campaigns and sanitation, play a vital role in preventing the spread of infectious diseases.
•   Scientific Advancements: Pandemics have driven scientific breakthroughs, from the discovery of bacteria and viruses to the development of vaccines and antiviral drugs.
•   Social Resilience: Societies have shown resilience and adaptability in the face of pandemics, leading to changes in governance, economics, and culture.
•   Global Cooperation: Addressing pandemics requires international cooperation and information sharing among nations.

Pandemics throughout history have been harrowing experiences, but they have also been catalysts for change. They have shaped the course of empires, influenced scientific and medical understanding, and altered the fabric of societies. While the human toll of pandemics is immense, the lessons learned from these historical events have helped us better prepare for and respond to future outbreaks. As we face the ongoing challenges of the COVID-19 pandemic and potential future threats, the wisdom gained from centuries of battling infectious diseases remains invaluable.

COVID-19: A Modern Case Study

The COVID-19 pandemic, caused by the novel coronavirus SARS-CoV-2, has been one of the most significant global health crises in recent history. This modern case study aims to delve into various aspects of the pandemic, ranging from its origins and spread to its impact on healthcare systems, economies, and society. As of my last knowledge update in September 2021, this comprehensive examination will provide a snapshot of our understanding and response up to that point.

I. The Emergence of SARS-CoV-2

The COVID-19 pandemic began with the emergence of a new coronavirus in Wuhan, China, in late 2019. The virus, initially referred to as the "Wuhan coronavirus" or "2019-nCoV," soon became known as SARS-CoV-2. Understanding the origin of the virus is crucial for preventing future pandemics.

A. Zoonotic Origins

•	SARS-CoV-2 is believed to have originated in bats and possibly passed through an intermediate host, such as a pangolin, before infecting humans. This zoonotic transmission highlights the interconnectedness of human and animal health.

B. Controversy Surrounding the Wuhan Institute of Virology

•	The Wuhan Institute of Virology, located in the city where the outbreak began, faced scrutiny regarding the possibility of a laboratory leak as the source of the virus. Investigations into this theory have been ongoing, emphasizing the need for transparency in global health research.

II. Global Spread and Response

The rapid spread of SARS-CoV-2 showcased the interconnectedness of our modern world and the challenges in containing a highly contagious virus.

A. Early Global Response

•	Many countries, including China, implemented strict lockdowns, travel restrictions, and quarantine measures to control the virus's spread. However, the virus had already begun its journey across borders.

B. The Role of the World Health Organization (WHO)

•   The WHO declared COVID-19 a pandemic in March 2020, highlighting the urgency of the situation. The organization played a critical role in coordinating international responses and providing guidance.

C. Vaccination Efforts

•   The development and distribution of COVID-19 vaccines represented a remarkable achievement of modern science. Multiple vaccines received emergency use authorization, but challenges in equitable distribution persist.

III. Impact on Healthcare Systems

COVID-19 placed immense strain on healthcare systems worldwide, exposing vulnerabilities and prompting adaptations.

A. Overwhelmed Hospitals

•   Hospitals faced overcrowding, shortages of personal protective equipment (PPE), and the need to adapt to a surge in critically ill patients. The situation highlighted the importance of healthcare system preparedness.

B. Telemedicine and Digital Health

•   The pandemic accelerated the adoption of telemedicine and digital health solutions, allowing for remote consultations and monitoring. This shift is likely to have lasting impacts on healthcare delivery.

C. Mental Health Crisis

•   The pandemic's toll on mental health became increasingly apparent, with rising rates of anxiety, depression, and other mental health issues. The need for mental health support and services gained recognition.

IV. Economic Consequences

The economic impact of COVID-19 has been profound, affecting industries, jobs, and government responses.

A. Economic Downturn

•	Lockdowns and reduced consumer activity led to recessions in many countries. Governments implemented stimulus packages to mitigate economic hardships.

B. The Rise of Remote Work

•	Remote work became the norm for many, leading to a reevaluation of traditional office-based work. This shift could have long-term implications for urban planning and the commercial real estate market.

C. Disparities Exposed

•	The pandemic disproportionately affected vulnerable populations and highlighted existing economic disparities. Addressing these inequalities became a focal point of recovery efforts.

V. Societal and Cultural Impacts

COVID-19 influenced every aspect of society, from how we interact with one another to the ways we view public health and government.

A. Changes in Behavior

•	Social distancing, mask-wearing, and increased hand hygiene became standard practices. These changes in behavior may persist long after the pandemic subsides.

B. Information and Misinformation

•	The infodemic, an overabundance of information, made it challenging to discern accurate information from falsehoods. Media literacy and science communication gained importance.

C. Trust in Institutions

•	Trust in governments, healthcare institutions, and scientific expertise became a central issue. Public perception of how authorities handled the crisis varied widely.

VI. Lessons Learned and Future Preparedness

The COVID-19 pandemic offers valuable lessons for how the world can better prepare for and respond to future health crises.

A. Global Collaboration

•   The pandemic underscored the need for international cooperation and information sharing to detect and respond to emerging threats.

B. Investment in Public Health

•   Governments recognized the importance of robust public health systems and the need for ongoing investment in disease surveillance, research, and healthcare infrastructure.

C. Pandemic Preparedness

•   The world is now more attuned to the potential for pandemics. Preparedness efforts, including vaccine research and development, have intensified.

COVID-19 serves as a modern case study in many facets of our interconnected world, from the emergence of infectious diseases to the response of governments, healthcare systems, and society at large. The pandemic has revealed both strengths and weaknesses in our global readiness to face such challenges. As of my last update in September 2021, the world was still grappling with the pandemic's effects, and the long-term impact remains uncertain. However, the lessons learned from this crisis will undoubtedly shape our approach to future health emergencies, underscoring the importance of global cooperation, scientific innovation, and societal resilience.

Part V: Response and Preparedness

Biological warfare, often referred to as biowarfare or germ warfare, is the deliberate use of biological agents, such as bacteria, viruses, or toxins, to cause harm to humans, animals, or plants. The use of biological agents as weapons has a long history dating back to ancient times, but it gained significant attention during the 20th century with the development of advanced technologies. In this article, we will explore the critical aspects of response and preparedness in the context of biological warfare.

Nature of Biological Warfare Agents

Biological warfare agents are unique in their ability to cause widespread harm through the transmission of diseases. They can be classified into several categories:

1.   Bacteria: Bacterial agents include pathogens like anthrax (Bacillus anthracis) and tularemia (Francisella tularensis). These agents can be weaponized and distributed through aerosols, food, or water, causing various diseases depending on the specific bacterium.
2.   Viruses: Viruses, such as smallpox or Ebola, are extremely contagious and can lead to devastating outbreaks when used as weapons. They are typically transmitted through respiratory droplets or bodily fluids.
3.   Toxins: Toxins like ricin or botulinum toxin are naturally produced by certain organisms. These toxins can be isolated and weaponized, leading to severe illness or death when introduced into a target population.

Historical Examples of Biological Warfare

1.   World War I: During World War I, both the Allied and Central Powers attempted to use biological agents, primarily bacteria, as weapons. However, these attempts were largely ineffective.
2.   World War II: Japan's Unit 731 conducted extensive research into biological warfare during World War II, using human subjects for experimentation. They dropped plague-infected fleas over Chinese cities, causing outbreaks.
3.   Cold War Era: The United States and the Soviet Union engaged in significant research and development of biological weapons during the Cold War. Fortunately, the Biological Weapons Convention (BWC) was established in 1972, which banned the production and use of biological weapons.

Response Strategies

Responding to a biological warfare attack is complex and challenging due to the invisible and often delayed nature of the threat. Effective response strategies must consider the following:

1.   Early Detection: Rapid identification of a biological attack is critical. Surveillance systems, both civilian and military, should be in place to detect unusual disease patterns or outbreaks.
2.   Isolation and Quarantine: Once a biological attack is confirmed, isolation and quarantine measures are crucial to prevent the spread of the disease. Infected individuals must be separated from the healthy population.
3.   Medical Countermeasures: Treatment and vaccination strategies should be readily available. Stockpiles of vaccines, antiviral drugs, and medical supplies are essential.
4.   Communication: Clear and accurate communication to the public is vital to prevent panic and ensure that individuals are informed about the situation and the necessary precautions.
5.   Coordination: Response efforts require close coordination between various agencies, including public health, law enforcement, and emergency management.
6.   Decontamination: Decontaminating affected areas is essential to remove biological agents and prevent further infection.
7.   Contact Tracing: Identifying and monitoring individuals who may have been exposed to the biological agent is critical to prevent secondary transmission.

Preparedness Measures

1.   Biological Threat Assessments: Governments and international organizations must continually assess the global biological threat landscape to understand potential risks and vulnerabilities.
2.   Research and Development: Investment in research and development of medical countermeasures, such as vaccines and treatments, is essential to stay ahead of evolving biological threats.
3.   Stockpiling: Maintaining stockpiles of vaccines, antibiotics, antiviral drugs, and personal protective equipment (PPE) is crucial for rapid response.
4.   Training and Exercises: Regular training and simulation exercises involving various response agencies help ensure that personnel are prepared to handle a biological attack effectively.
5.   International Cooperation: Collaborative efforts between countries are essential to share information, intelligence, and resources to respond to transnational biological threats.

Biological warfare presents a unique and challenging threat to global security. Responding effectively to such an attack requires early detection, rapid response, and close coordination among various agencies. Preparedness measures, including research and development, stockpiling, and international cooperation, are essential to mitigate the risks associated with biological warfare. In an increasingly interconnected world, the importance of a robust response and preparedness framework cannot be overstated in safeguarding the health and security of nations.

Biosecurity and Biosafety

In the modern age, advancements in science and technology have ushered in unprecedented opportunities and challenges. As we delve deeper into understanding the complexities of life, our ability to manipulate and control biological systems has grown exponentially. However, this newfound power comes with significant responsibilities. Biosecurity and biosafety have emerged as critical fields of study and practice, aimed at safeguarding life forms, ecosystems, and human society from the potential risks associated with advances in biology and biotechnology.

This comprehensive exploration of biosecurity and biosafety will delve into the fundamental concepts, historical context, regulatory frameworks, emerging challenges, and the ethical considerations that shape these domains. By the end of this discussion, we will have a comprehensive understanding of the intricate interplay between science, ethics, and policy in the realm of biosecurity and biosafety.

I. Fundamental Concepts

1.1. Biosecurity vs. Biosafety: Distinguishing Terminology

Biosecurity and biosafety are two closely related but distinct concepts that underpin the safety and security of biological research, technologies, and materials. Understanding the differences between these terms is crucial for navigating the complex landscape of biotechnology governance.

Biosecurity primarily pertains to the protection of biological materials, technologies, and information from theft, loss, or intentional misuse for harmful purposes. It encompasses measures to prevent unauthorized access to, theft of, or tampering with biological agents or materials. In essence, biosecurity focuses on safeguarding against the intentional misuse of biological resources.

Biosafety, on the other hand, revolves around the safe handling, containment, and management of biological materials to protect researchers, the environment, and the public from accidental exposure to potential hazards. It deals with preventing unintentional harm that may arise during laboratory research, manufacturing processes, or the handling of biological materials.

1.2. Historical Perspective

The roots of biosecurity and biosafety can be traced back to some of the darkest chapters in human history. The use of biological agents as weapons dates back centuries, with instances like the deliberate distribution of smallpox-infected blankets to Native Americans by European settlers. These early examples highlight the potential for bioweapons to cause widespread harm.

The horrors of World War I and World War II brought the issue of biological weapons to the forefront of global consciousness. The Geneva Protocol of 1925 banned the use of biological weapons in warfare, marking the first international attempt to address biosecurity concerns. However, it wasn't until the Biological Weapons Convention (BWC) of 1972 that a comprehensive treaty was established to prohibit the development, production, and acquisition of biological weapons.

The emergence of modern biotechnology in the latter half of the 20th century presented both incredible opportunities for scientific progress and new challenges in biosecurity and biosafety. As genetic engineering and biotechnology advanced, so did the need for robust safeguards against unintended consequences and misuse.

II. Regulatory Frameworks

2.1. International Agreements

The international community has recognized the importance of global cooperation in addressing biosecurity and biosafety concerns. The Biological Weapons Convention (BWC) remains a cornerstone of international efforts to prevent the use of biological weapons. Under the BWC, signatory states commit to prohibiting the development and use of biological weapons and to promoting peaceful uses of biological science and technology.

The Convention on Biological Diversity (CBD) is another significant international agreement that addresses the conservation of biodiversity and the sustainable use of biological resources. While not primarily focused on biosecurity, the CBD indirectly influences efforts to protect ecosystems and prevent the spread of invasive species, which are essential aspects of biosafety.

2.2. National Regulations

At the national level, countries develop their own regulatory frameworks for biosecurity and biosafety. These frameworks can vary widely in scope and stringency. Regulatory agencies, such as the United States Centers for Disease Control and Prevention (CDC) and the U.S. Department of Agriculture (USDA), oversee biosafety and biosecurity measures in the United States.

In many countries, research involving potentially hazardous biological materials is subject to stringent oversight, with researchers required to adhere to specific containment protocols and reporting requirements. This ensures that research is conducted safely and transparently.

2.3. Laboratory Biosafety Levels

Laboratories are categorized into biosafety levels (BSL) based on the level of containment required for the research being conducted. The World Health Organization (WHO) has established guidelines for BSLs, ranging from BSL-1 (minimal risk) to BSL-4 (highest containment). BSL-4 laboratories are equipped to handle the most dangerous pathogens, such as Ebola and Marburg viruses.

These containment levels dictate the physical infrastructure, safety procedures, and personnel training necessary to safely conduct research involving various biological agents. Maintaining these containment levels is essential to prevent accidental releases or exposure to hazardous materials.

III. Emerging Challenges

3.1. Dual-Use Dilemma

One of the most pressing challenges in biosecurity is the dual-use dilemma. Dual-use research refers to scientific studies that have both beneficial and harmful applications. While research may be conducted with the intent of advancing medical or scientific knowledge, the same findings could potentially be exploited for malevolent purposes.

For example, studies on the genetic modification of pathogens to understand their virulence could inadvertently provide insights into how to enhance their lethality. Striking a balance between enabling scientific progress and preventing misuse is a complex ethical and policy challenge.

3.2. Synthetic Biology and Gene Editing

The advent of synthetic biology and powerful gene-editing techniques like CRISPR-Cas9 has amplified biosecurity concerns. These technologies allow for the design and modification of biological systems with unprecedented precision. While they hold immense promise for medicine, agriculture, and industry, they also raise fears about the creation of novel, potentially harmful organisms or the manipulation of existing ones for nefarious purposes.

The case of gene drive technology, which can rapidly spread engineered genes through populations, exemplifies the biosecurity and biosafety challenges posed by synthetic biology. There are concerns that gene drives could be used to alter or eliminate entire species, with unpredictable consequences for ecosystems.

3.3. Cyberbiosecurity

As biological research becomes increasingly reliant on digital data and automation, the field of cyberbiosecurity has emerged. Cyberbiosecurity deals with protecting the integrity and security of biological data, laboratory equipment, and systems. This includes safeguarding against cyberattacks that could manipulate or compromise biological research.

For instance, a cyberattack on a biomanufacturing facility could disrupt the production of critical medical supplies or even lead to the accidental release of hazardous materials. Ensuring robust cybersecurity measures in the life sciences sector is essential to prevent such risks.

IV. Ethical Considerations

4.1. Ethical Dilemmas in Dual-Use Research

The ethical dilemmas surrounding dual-use research are multifaceted. Researchers and institutions must grapple with questions of scientific freedom, censorship, and the potential harm that could result from their work. Striking a balance between openness and responsible conduct is challenging but crucial.

Ethical frameworks, such as the Asilomar Guidelines for Recombinant DNA Research, have been developed to guide researchers in navigating these complex issues. These guidelines emphasize transparency, risk assessment, and ethical review to ensure that research benefits outweigh potential harms.

4.2. Access to Benefits vs. Security

Balancing access to the benefits of biotechnology with security concerns is another ethical challenge. Access to life-saving medical treatments, improved agricultural practices, and sustainable bioenergy sources must be equitable. However, the fear of misuse often leads to restrictive policies that can hinder the global distribution of beneficial technologies. Striking a balance between promoting scientific collaboration and safeguarding against misuse is a continuous ethical and policy struggle.

4.3. Environmental and Ecological Ethics

Biosafety extends beyond the laboratory to encompass the broader environment and ecosystems. Genetic modification of organisms for agricultural or environmental purposes raises ethical questions about unintended consequences. For instance, genetically modified crops resistant to pests may inadvertently harm non-target species, disrupt ecosystems, or create unforeseen ecological imbalances.

The precautionary principle, which suggests that when an activity raises threats of harm to the environment, precautionary measures should be taken, is often invoked in these situations. Ethical considerations in biosafety necessitate comprehensive risk assessments and ecological monitoring to minimize harm to the environment.

4.4. Equity and Global Governance

Access to advanced biotechnology and the benefits it offers is not evenly distributed across the globe. Ethical concerns arise regarding the disparities in resources, knowledge, and capabilities between developed and developing nations. Global governance mechanisms must address these disparities to ensure that biosecurity and biosafety efforts are equitable and inclusive.

Efforts such as the Nagoya Protocol under the Convention on Biological Diversity aim to promote the fair and equitable sharing of benefits arising from the utilization of genetic resources. Ethical discussions surrounding global governance emphasize the importance of respecting the sovereignty of nations while fostering international cooperation.

V. Case Studies

5.1. The Anthrax Attacks of 2001

The anthrax attacks in the United States in 2001 serve as a chilling reminder of the biosecurity challenges the world faces. Letters containing anthrax spores were sent to various media outlets and government offices, resulting in the deaths of five people and several others falling ill. This incident highlighted the potential for bioterrorism and the need for robust biosecurity measures to prevent unauthorized access to dangerous biological agents.

Investigations into the source of the anthrax used in the attacks underscored the importance of traceability and security in handling biological materials. The case also spurred improvements in laboratory security protocols and national preparedness for bioterrorism threats.

5.2. The CRISPR Babies Scandal

In 2018, Chinese scientist He Jiankui claimed to have created the world's first genetically edited babies using CRISPR-Cas9 technology. He's actions raised profound ethical concerns as he had not followed established ethical and regulatory guidelines. The experiment's lack of transparency, informed consent, and thorough risk assessment sparked international outrage and renewed discussions on the ethical boundaries of gene editing.

The scandal highlighted the importance of responsible conduct in research and the need for clear regulatory frameworks to govern the use of powerful gene-editing tools like CRISPR-Cas9. It also underscored the urgency of addressing ethical concerns related to human germline editing.

VI. Future Directions

6.1. Strengthening Global Cooperation

As biotechnology continues to advance, global cooperation in biosecurity and biosafety becomes increasingly vital. International collaboration on surveillance, information sharing, and capacity building is essential to detect and respond to emerging threats promptly.

Efforts like the Global Health Security Agenda (GHSA) and the Global Initiative to Combat Nuclear Terrorism (GICNT) exemplify international initiatives aimed at enhancing biosecurity preparedness. Strengthening these partnerships and expanding their scope is essential for addressing evolving challenges.

6.2. Ethical Frameworks and Guidelines

The development of ethical frameworks and guidelines remains a crucial aspect of biosecurity and biosafety. Ethical considerations should be integrated into research practices and policy decisions to ensure responsible conduct in science and technology.

Engaging scientists, ethicists, policymakers, and the public in ongoing dialogues about the ethical implications of biotechnology will help navigate the complexities of dual-use research, equitable access, and environmental protection.

6.3. Emerging Technologies and Preparedness

As emerging technologies like synthetic biology and gene editing continue to evolve, biosecurity and biosafety measures must keep pace. Research institutions and governments should invest in research and development of new tools and strategies to mitigate risks associated with these technologies.

Additionally, preparedness and response plans for bioterrorism and infectious disease outbreaks should be regularly updated and tested to ensure effective responses in times of crisis.

In an era defined by unprecedented scientific progress and technological innovation, biosecurity and biosafety are essential components of responsible research and innovation. These fields aim to strike a delicate balance between advancing knowledge, promoting global equity, and safeguarding against the misuse of biotechnology.

The history of biosecurity and biosafety reveals the lessons learned from past mistakes, from the horrors of bioweapons to the challenges of genetic editing. Today, the world faces complex challenges in the form of dual-use research, synthetic biology, and cyberbiosecurity.

Ethical considerations permeate every aspect of biosecurity and biosafety, guiding researchers, policymakers, and society as they grapple with these complex issues. Balancing scientific freedom with responsible conduct, ensuring equitable access to benefits, and protecting the environment are paramount concerns.

As we move forward into an uncertain future filled with the promise and peril of biotechnology, it is our collective responsibility to prioritize the safety and security of life in all its forms. By strengthening international cooperation, adhering to ethical principles, and embracing emerging technologies with caution and responsibility, we can navigate the intricate terrain of biosecurity and biosafety while fostering a world where science serves the betterment of humanity.

Laboratory Safety

Laboratories are the bedrock of scientific discovery and technological advancement. They serve as the crucible where researchers and scientists unravel the mysteries of the natural world, develop life-saving drugs, engineer groundbreaking technologies, and conduct a myriad of experiments that shape our understanding of the universe. However, the very nature of laboratories, with their potent chemicals, high-energy equipment, and complex processes, presents inherent risks to those who work within their confines. Therefore, laboratory safety is not merely a regulatory requirement; it is a moral and ethical imperative.

In this comprehensive exploration of laboratory safety, we will delve into the importance of laboratory safety, examine the risks and hazards present in laboratories, discuss the key principles and guidelines for safe laboratory practices, and explore how modern technologies and methodologies are enhancing laboratory safety.

Chapter 1: The Importance of Laboratory Safety

1.1. Protecting Lives

Laboratory safety is paramount for the protection of human lives. Laboratories house a plethora of hazardous materials, ranging from corrosive chemicals to flammable substances and biological agents. Mishandling or improper storage of these materials can lead to accidents, injuries, or even fatalities. The tragic consequences of lax safety measures underscore the critical importance of prioritizing safety in laboratories.

1.2. Preservation of Scientific Integrity

Safety is not merely about preventing accidents; it also ensures the integrity of scientific experiments and data. Contamination, equipment malfunction, or accidents can compromise the validity of research results, rendering months or years of work futile. By adhering to rigorous safety protocols, scientists uphold the credibility of their work and maintain the trust of the scientific community.

1.3. Legal and Ethical Responsibilities

Laboratory safety is not a matter of choice; it is a legal and ethical obligation. Governments, regulatory agencies, and institutions have established stringent regulations and guidelines to safeguard laboratory personnel, the environment, and the public. Non-compliance with these regulations can result in legal repercussions, fines, or the shutdown of laboratories.

Chapter 2: Risks and Hazards in Laboratories

2.1. Chemical Hazards

One of the most prevalent risks in laboratories comes from the chemicals used in experiments. These hazards include corrosive chemicals that can cause burns, toxic substances that can lead to poisoning, and flammable materials that can cause fires or explosions. The improper handling, storage, or disposal of chemicals can have dire consequences.

2.2. Biological Hazards

Biological laboratories deal with living organisms, including bacteria, viruses, and fungi. Exposure to these agents can lead to infections and illnesses. Proper containment, personal protective equipment (PPE), and strict adherence to biosafety protocols are essential to mitigate these risks.

2.3. Radiation Hazards

Laboratories utilizing radiation sources, such as X-rays or radioactive materials, pose unique risks. Unprotected exposure to ionizing radiation can result in severe health consequences, including radiation sickness and an increased risk of cancer. Shielding, monitoring, and strict protocols are crucial to minimize radiation hazards.

2.4. Physical Hazards

Laboratories often house equipment that can be physically hazardous. High-speed centrifuges, high-pressure reactors, and electrical apparatus can pose risks of mechanical injuries, electrical shocks, or explosions if not operated correctly.

2.5. Fire and Explosion Hazards

The presence of flammable chemicals, compressed gases, and electrical equipment creates an environment susceptible to fires and explosions. Laboratory safety measures include fire-resistant construction, fire extinguishers, and fire evacuation plans.

2.6. Ergonomic and Psychosocial Hazards

Beyond the immediate physical dangers, laboratories can also pose ergonomic and psychosocial risks. Prolonged exposure to uncomfortable workstations or the pressure of meeting tight deadlines can lead to stress, fatigue, and musculoskeletal disorders.

Chapter 3: Principles of Laboratory Safety

3.1. Risk Assessment

The foundation of laboratory safety is the assessment of risks associated with specific experiments or procedures. Scientists and researchers must identify potential hazards, evaluate their likelihood and severity, and implement controls to mitigate these risks.

3.2. Training and Education

Laboratory personnel should receive comprehensive training in laboratory safety practices. This includes understanding the hazards present, proper handling of equipment and materials, and emergency response procedures. Ongoing education is vital to stay current with safety protocols.

3.3. Personal Protective Equipment (PPE)

The use of appropriate PPE, such as lab coats, gloves, safety goggles, and respirators, is non-negotiable. PPE serves as the last line of defense against chemical spills, biological contamination, and physical hazards.

3.4. Standard Operating Procedures (SOPs)

Laboratories should establish and enforce SOPs for every experiment and procedure. These SOPs detail step-by-step instructions, safety precautions, and emergency response measures, ensuring consistency and safety across all activities.

3.5. Engineering Controls

Engineering controls involve the design of laboratory facilities and equipment to minimize risks. Examples include fume hoods to contain chemical fumes, safety interlocks on machinery, and ventilation systems to remove harmful gases.

3.6. Emergency Response Plans

Laboratories must have well-defined emergency response plans in place. These plans cover actions to take in the event of fires, chemical spills, injuries, or other emergencies. Regular drills and training ensure readiness.

Chapter 4: Advancements in Laboratory Safety

4.1. Automation and Robotics

Automation and robotics are transforming laboratory safety by reducing the need for human intervention in high-risk processes. Automated systems can handle dangerous chemicals, perform repetitive tasks, and provide consistent results while keeping researchers out of harm's way.

4.2. Sensor Technologies

The integration of advanced sensors in laboratories enhances safety by continuously monitoring conditions such as temperature, pressure, gas levels, and radiation. Real-time data and alarms help prevent accidents and provide early warnings.

4.3. Data Analytics and Machine Learning

Data analytics and machine learning algorithms analyze laboratory data to detect patterns and anomalies. These technologies can identify potential safety hazards, predict equipment failures, and optimize safety protocols based on historical data.

4.4. Virtual and Augmented Reality

Virtual and augmented reality technologies enable researchers to conduct experiments in simulated environments, reducing the risks associated with physical experimentation. This approach allows for training, testing, and troubleshooting without exposure to actual hazards.

4.5. Remote Monitoring and Control

Remote monitoring and control systems allow researchers to oversee experiments and equipment from a safe distance. This minimizes the need for direct physical presence in high-risk environments, reducing the potential for accidents.

Chapter 5: Case Studies in Laboratory Safety

5.1. Chernobyl Nuclear Disaster

The Chernobyl nuclear disaster in 1986 serves as a haunting reminder of the catastrophic consequences of lax safety practices. A combination of design flaws, operator errors, and inadequate safety protocols resulted in a massive radioactive release, leading to immediate deaths, long-term health effects, and environmental devastation.

5.2. Bhopal Gas Tragedy

The Bhopal gas tragedy in 1984 was one of the world's worst industrial disasters. A gas leak from a pesticide plant exposed thousands of people to toxic methyl isocyanate gas, resulting in thousands of deaths and long-term health issues. Inadequate safety measures and poor maintenance were primary factors in this tragedy.

5.3. Space Shuttle Challenger Disaster

The Space Shuttle Challenger disaster in 1986 was a sobering lesson in the importance of thorough safety checks. A flawed O-ring seal in one of the solid rocket boosters led to the shuttle's explosion shortly after liftoff , resulting in the tragic deaths of all seven crew members. This disaster underscored the necessity of rigorous safety inspections and the importance of whistleblowers who raise concerns about potential hazards.

5.4. SARS-CoV-2 Research and Laboratory Safety

The COVID-19 pandemic brought laboratory safety into the spotlight. Research laboratories worldwide raced to study the SARS-CoV-2 virus and develop vaccines. Proper containment and safety measures were crucial to prevent accidental exposures to the virus. Labs conducting this research had to adhere to strict biosafety protocols to protect researchers and prevent the virus from escaping into the community.

These case studies serve as poignant reminders of the catastrophic consequences that can result from negligence or inadequate safety measures in laboratories. They highlight the need for continuous vigilance and the implementation of the highest safety standards in all scientific endeavors.

Chapter 6: Ethical Considerations in Laboratory Safety

6.1. Accountability and Responsibility

Scientists and researchers bear a profound ethical responsibility for the safety of themselves, their colleagues, and the broader community. This includes following safety protocols, reporting hazards, and refusing to engage in research or experiments that they believe pose undue risks.

6.2. Transparency and Disclosure

Transparent communication of potential risks associated with research is essential. This extends to informing participants in clinical trials or studies about the risks involved and obtaining informed consent. Transparency also applies to sharing safety data and lessons learned with the scientific community.

6.3. Balancing Scientific Progress and Safety

The pursuit of scientific progress should never come at the expense of safety. Ethical dilemmas can arise when researchers face pressure to advance their work quickly. Balancing the need for innovation with safety considerations is a fundamental ethical challenge.

6.4. Whistleblower Protection

Whistleblowers play a critical role in identifying safety violations or ethical misconduct in laboratories. Ethical considerations demand that institutions protect whistleblowers from retaliation and ensure their concerns are thoroughly investigated.

Chapter 7: Regulatory Framework for Laboratory Safety

7.1. Occupational Safety and Health Administration (OSHA)

In the United States, OSHA sets and enforces workplace safety and health standards. OSHA's regulations cover a wide range of laboratory activities, from chemical handling to electrical safety, and require employers to provide training, PPE, and hazard communication.

7.2. Environmental Protection Agency (EPA)

The EPA regulates the handling and disposal of hazardous chemicals and waste in laboratories. Laboratories must comply with EPA regulations to protect the environment and public health.

7.3. Biosafety and Biosecurity Regulations

For laboratories working with biological agents, the CDC and NIH in the United States, as well as international organizations like the World Health Organization (WHO), provide guidelines and regulations to ensure safe handling and containment of biological materials.

7.4. International Standards

Laboratory safety is a global concern, and international standards such as ISO 45001 for occupational health and safety management systems provide a framework for organizations worldwide to improve safety practices.

Chapter 8: Future Trends and Challenges in Laboratory Safety

8.1. Emerging Technologies

As laboratories continue to evolve with advancements in science and technology, new risks and challenges emerge. The integration of nanotechnology, synthetic biology, and artificial intelligence in research introduces novel safety considerations that require careful management.

8.2. Cross-Disciplinary Collaboration

Interdisciplinary research brings together experts from diverse fields, each with their own safety protocols and practices. Ensuring a cohesive safety culture across disciplines is a challenge that requires effective communication and collaboration.

8.3. Public Awareness and Engagement

Laboratories are not isolated from the communities they inhabit. Building public trust and awareness about laboratory safety practices and research conducted in their vicinity is essential to maintaining harmonious relationships.

8.4. Cybersecurity Risks

Laboratories increasingly rely on digital infrastructure and connectivity, making them vulnerable to cyberattacks. Protecting sensitive data and ensuring the security of research infrastructure is a growing concern.

Laboratory safety is the cornerstone of scientific progress and ethical responsibility. The risks and hazards inherent in laboratories demand unwavering commitment to safety principles, rigorous adherence to regulations, and the integration of cutting-edge technologies to mitigate risks. The lessons learned from tragic incidents like Chernobyl, Bhopal, and Challenger underscore the imperative of maintaining the highest safety standards in all scientific endeavors.

As laboratories continue to push the boundaries of human knowledge and innovation, the pursuit of scientific progress must always be accompanied by an unwavering commitment to safeguarding lives, protecting the environment, and upholding the principles of ethical research. In doing so, we can ensure that laboratories remain the crucible of discovery, where the boundaries of human knowledge are pushed, and where safety is paramount in every experiment and exploration.

Dual-Use Research Concerns

Dual-use research concerns have become a focal point in the world of science and technology. The term "dual-use" refers to research that has the potential for both beneficial and harmful applications. While scientific progress has led to significant advancements in various fields, it has also raised ethical, safety, and security issues. This article delves into the multifaceted nature of dual-use research, its implications, and the measures taken to strike a balance between innovation and security.

I. The Dual-Use Dilemma

1.1. Defining Dual-Use Research

Dual-use research encompasses scientific investigations, experiments, or technological developments that can have dual, contrasting outcomes: one that benefits society and another that poses risks or harm. Such research can be found across various disciplines, including biology, chemistry, physics, and information technology.

1.2. Examples of Dual-Use Research

To illustrate the concept of dual-use research, let's consider some notable examples:

1.2.1. Biotechnology: Advances in biotechnology can lead to life-saving medical treatments, but they can also be employed for the creation of biological weapons.

1.2.2. Artificial Intelligence: AI systems have the potential to revolutionize industries, but they can also be misused for deepfake videos or autonomous weaponry.

1.2.3. Nuclear Science: Nuclear technology can provide clean energy, but it also has the potential for nuclear weapons development.

1.2.4. Information Security: Techniques used to protect data and networks can be used to safeguard information but also for cyberattacks and espionage.

1.3. Ethical Dimensions

The dual-use dilemma raises significant ethical questions. Scientists and researchers must consider not only the potential benefits of their work but also the potential harm it may cause. This ethical responsibility becomes particularly important when the risks are grave, as in the case of bioterrorism or nuclear proliferation.

II. Balancing Innovation and Security

2.1. The Need for Dual-Use Research

It's important to acknowledge that dual-use research isn't inherently negative. In many cases, it leads to groundbreaking innovations that benefit society. For example, the development of the internet, initially conceived for military communication, has transformed how the world connects and shares information.

2.2. Security Concerns

However, the proliferation of dual-use research also comes with security concerns. Rogue actors, whether state-sponsored or independent, can exploit scientific advancements for malicious purposes. This has led to a delicate balancing act between promoting innovation and protecting national and global security.

2.3. Regulatory Measures

To address dual-use research concerns, governments and international organizations have established regulatory measures. These include export controls, technology transfer restrictions, and guidelines for responsible conduct in research. The Biological Weapons Convention (BWC) and the Chemical Weapons Convention (CWC) are examples of international treaties aimed at preventing the misuse of scientific research.

III. The Life Sciences and Dual-Use Research

3.1. Biosecurity Threats

One of the most pressing dual-use concerns lies within the life sciences. Advances in biotechnology and genetic engineering have unlocked incredible potential for medical breakthroughs. However, these same technologies can also be employed to create dangerous pathogens or bioweapons.

3.2. The Gain-of-Function Debate

The gain-of-function (GoF) debate exemplifies the complexity of dual-use research in the life sciences. GoF experiments involve enhancing the virulence, transmissibility, or host range of pathogens to understand their potential risks. Critics argue that these experiments could inadvertently create a more dangerous pathogen, while proponents claim they are essential for preparedness and vaccine development.

3.3. Controversial Experiments

In recent years, controversial experiments, such as the creation of a more transmissible H5N1 avian influenza virus, have sparked intense debates. These controversies have led to calls for stricter oversight and evaluation of dual-use research projects.

IV. Ethical Considerations and Dual-Use Research

4.1. The Responsibility of Scientists

Scientists engaged in dual-use research face a moral dilemma. They must strike a balance between advancing knowledge and ensuring the responsible use of their findings. This requires self-regulation, transparency, and collaboration with oversight bodies.

4.2. Open Science vs. Security

The principle of open science, which advocates for the unrestricted sharing of research findings, can clash with security concerns related to dual-use research. Striking the right balance between openness and security remains a challenge.

V. Safeguarding Against Dual-Use Research Risks

5.1. Biosecurity Measures

Efforts to mitigate the risks of dual-use research include enhancing biosecurity measures within laboratories. This involves strict access controls, personnel screening, and secure storage of dangerous materials.

5.2. Education and Awareness

Raising awareness among scientists and researchers about the dual-use dilemma is essential. Educational programs can help scientists understand their ethical responsibilities and the potential consequences of their work.

5.3. International Collaboration

Collaboration between countries is crucial in addressing dual-use research concerns. International agreements and information sharing can help prevent the misuse of scientific knowledge.

VI. Case Studies

6.1. The 2001 Anthrax Attacks

The 2001 anthrax attacks in the United States highlighted the dual-use potential of biotechnology. Anthrax spores were weaponized and sent through the mail, resulting in multiple deaths. This event underscored the need for heightened biosecurity measures.

6.2. Cybersecurity Threats

The realm of information technology is also fraught with dual-use concerns. Cyberattacks, driven by state and non-state actors, leverage advanced technology for espionage and disruption. This has led to ongoing debates about the responsible use of cybersecurity research.

VII. The Future of Dual-Use Research

7.1. Emerging Technologies

As science and technology continue to advance, new dual-use concerns will emerge. Emerging fields like quantum computing, synthetic biology, and space exploration present unique challenges that require proactive risk assessment and regulation.

7.2. International Cooperation

The global nature of dual-use research necessitates international cooperation. Countries must work together to establish common guidelines and best practices to prevent misuse while fostering scientific progress.

7.3. Ethical Frameworks

Developing robust ethical frameworks for evaluating dual-use research projects will be essential. These frameworks should consider both the potential benefits and risks associated with scientific advancements.

Dual-use research concerns are an intrinsic part of the ever-evolving landscape of science and technology. Balancing innovation and security in this context is an ongoing challenge that requires collaboration, responsible conduct, and ethical reflection. As we continue to push the boundaries of knowledge, it is imperative that we remain vigilant and proactive in addressing the ethical and security dimensions of dual-use research.

Only through such efforts can we harness the full potential of scientific advancement while safeguarding against its darker consequences.

Epidemic and Pandemic Preparedness

Epidemics and pandemics have been an integral part of human history for centuries. From the Black Death in the 14th century to the Spanish flu in the 20th century, infectious diseases have repeatedly ravaged populations across the globe. The COVID-19 pandemic, which began in 2019, brought the world to a standstill and underscored the importance of effective epidemic and pandemic preparedness. In this comprehensive essay, we will explore the concepts of epidemic and pandemic preparedness, their historical context, the lessons learned from past outbreaks, and the strategies and measures necessary to mitigate the impact of future infectious disease threats.

Historical Context

Throughout history, epidemics and pandemics have caused immense suffering and shaped the course of human societies. The Black Death, which struck Europe in the 14th century, is estimated to have wiped out one-third of the European population. It serves as a grim reminder of the devastating potential of infectious diseases in a world with limited medical knowledge and resources.

Fast forward to the 20th century, and we encounter the Spanish flu of 1918-1919, which infected a third of the world's population and claimed the lives of approximately 50 million people. The world was ill-prepared to combat this influenza pandemic, highlighting the need for a coordinated global response.

The more recent epidemics, such as the HIV/AIDS crisis in the 1980s and 1990s and the Ebola outbreaks in West Africa in the 2010s, have further underscored the importance of preparedness, rapid response, and international collaboration in tackling infectious diseases.

Lessons from Past Epidemics and Pandemics

1.   Surveillance and Early Detection: One of the most critical lessons from past outbreaks is the importance of early detection and surveillance. Timely identification of cases and tracking of the disease's spread can significantly mitigate its impact. The use of modern technology, including real-time data analysis and monitoring, has revolutionized surveillance efforts.
2.   Vaccine Development: The development and distribution of vaccines have been instrumental in controlling and preventing epidemics. The smallpox eradication campaign, led by the World Health Organization (WHO), serves as a model for successful global vaccination efforts. The rapid development of COVID-19 vaccines in

record time further highlights the potential of science and innovation in epidemic response.

3.   Healthcare Infrastructure: A robust healthcare infrastructure is essential in managing epidemics. This includes having adequate hospital beds, medical supplies, and trained healthcare professionals. The shortage of ventilators and personal protective equipment (PPE) during the COVID-19 pandemic exposed vulnerabilities in healthcare systems worldwide.

4.   Public Health Measures: Non-pharmaceutical interventions, such as social distancing, mask-wearing, and quarantine measures, have proven effective in slowing the spread of infectious diseases. Public compliance with these measures is crucial for epidemic control.

5.   International Cooperation: Epidemics and pandemics do not respect borders. International cooperation and information-sharing are vital for a coordinated response. Organizations like the WHO play a central role in facilitating global collaboration during health crises.

Strategies for Epidemic and Pandemic Preparedness

1.   Risk Assessment and Monitoring: Continuous risk assessment is essential to identify potential threats. Surveillance systems should be established to monitor outbreaks at the local, national, and international levels. Early warning systems can provide alerts for emerging diseases.

2.   Research and Development: Investment in research and development for vaccines, therapeutics, and diagnostics is crucial. Governments, pharmaceutical companies, and international organizations must work together to accelerate the development of medical countermeasures.

3.   Healthcare Infrastructure Strengthening: Building and maintaining a resilient healthcare infrastructure is paramount. This includes expanding hospital capacity, ensuring a steady supply of essential medical equipment and medications, and training healthcare workers in epidemic response protocols.

4.   Stockpiling: Maintaining strategic stockpiles of essential medical supplies, including PPE, antiviral medications, and vaccines, can ensure a rapid response to emerging epidemics. However, stockpiles must be regularly updated and rotated to prevent wastage.

5.   Public Health Education: Public awareness and education campaigns can promote good hygiene practices, vaccination, and compliance with public health measures. Effective communication can dispel misinformation and reduce panic during outbreaks.

6.   International Collaboration: Strengthening international collaboration through organizations like the WHO is vital. Countries must work together to share data, coordinate responses, and provide assistance to nations in need during epidemics.

7.   Contingency Planning: Governments and organizations should develop comprehensive contingency plans for epidemics and pandemics. These plans should outline roles, responsibilities, and procedures for responding to different scenarios.

8.   Community Engagement: Engaging with communities and respecting cultural sensitivities is essential for effective epidemic response. Communities can be valuable partners in contact tracing and disease control efforts.

Challenges and Barriers

While the strategies outlined above are essential for epidemic and pandemic preparedness, several challenges and barriers must be addressed:

1.   Global Inequality: Health systems in low-income countries often lack the resources and infrastructure needed to respond effectively to epidemics. Addressing global health inequality is crucial for a coordinated global response.

2.   Vaccine Distribution: Ensuring equitable access to vaccines remains a challenge. Vaccine nationalism and supply chain disruptions can hinder the timely distribution of vaccines to all regions of the world.

3.   Misinformation: The spread of misinformation and vaccine hesitancy can undermine public health efforts. Combatting false information and promoting trust in public health authorities are ongoing challenges.

4.   Political Interference: Political considerations can sometimes interfere with the transparent and evidence-based response to epidemics. Maintaining the independence and integrity of public health agencies is essential.

5.   Antimicrobial Resistance: The rise of antimicrobial resistance threatens our ability to treat infectious diseases. Addressing this challenge requires a global effort to steward antibiotics and develop new therapies.

Epidemic and pandemic preparedness are not optional but imperative for safeguarding global health and security. The lessons learned from past outbreaks underscore the importance of early detection, international collaboration, healthcare infrastructure, and public health measures. By implementing comprehensive strategies and addressing existing challenges, the world can better prepare for and respond to future epidemics and pandemics. As the COVID-19 pandemic has demonstrated, the stakes are high, and the consequences of inaction are devastating. It is our collective responsibility to prioritize epidemic and pandemic preparedness to protect the health and well-being of all people.

International Cooperation and Strategies

In a rapidly globalizing world, international cooperation has become paramount for addressing complex global challenges. Whether it's tackling climate change, responding to pandemics, promoting peace and security, or fostering economic growth, nations must work together to achieve common goals. This essay explores the significance of international cooperation and the strategies employed by countries and international organizations to foster collaboration in this interconnected world.

The Importance of International Cooperation

International cooperation is the foundation upon which the modern world order is built. It enables nations to pool resources, knowledge, and expertise to confront shared challenges. Here are some key reasons why international cooperation is essential:

1.   Global Challenges: Many of the most pressing issues facing humanity today, such as climate change, terrorism, and pandemics, transcend national borders. Solving these challenges requires collective action.
2.   Peace and Security: International cooperation, particularly through organizations like the United Nations, plays a vital role in preventing conflicts and maintaining peace among nations.
3.   Economic Interdependence: In an era of globalization, economies are highly interconnected. Nations must cooperate to ensure stable trade, investment, and economic growth.
4.   Humanitarian Aid: When natural disasters or humanitarian crises strike, international cooperation is crucial for delivering timely and effective aid to those in need.
5.   Technological Advancement: Scientific and technological progress often relies on collaboration between countries, as seen in the development of the International Space Station or collaborative research in particle physics.

Now that we've established the importance of international cooperation, let's delve into the strategies employed to facilitate it.

Strategies for International Cooperation

1.   Diplomacy: Diplomacy is the art of conducting negotiations between nations. Diplomatic channels are essential for resolving disputes, forging alliances, and reaching agreements. Embassies, ambassadors, and international summits serve as crucial instruments of diplomacy.

2.   International Treaties and Agreements: Nations formalize their commitment to cooperation through treaties and agreements. Examples include the Paris Agreement on climate change, the United Nations Charter, and numerous trade agreements like NAFTA (North American Free Trade Agreement).

3.   Multilateral Organizations: International organizations, such as the United Nations, World Trade Organization (WTO), and World Health Organization (WHO), facilitate cooperation among multiple nations. These organizations provide forums for discussions, coordination, and dispute resolution.

4.   Bilateral Relations: Countries often build strong bilateral relations with key partners. These close ties can lead to more effective cooperation on various issues, from trade agreements to joint research projects.

5.   Soft Power and Cultural Diplomacy: Soft power, a term coined by Joseph Nye, refers to a nation's ability to influence others through culture, values, and ideas rather than coercion or force. Cultural diplomacy, such as promoting a nation's language, arts, and education, can help build positive relationships with other countries.

6.   Economic Cooperation: Economic collaboration, through organizations like the International Monetary Fund (IMF) or the World Bank, is crucial for stabilizing financial systems and fostering economic growth worldwide.

7.   Security Alliances: Countries form security alliances, such as NATO (North Atlantic Treaty Organization), to enhance their collective defense against common threats. These alliances create deterrence and promote stability.

8.   Development Assistance: Developed nations often provide aid and development assistance to less-developed countries. These programs aim to reduce poverty, improve healthcare and education, and promote sustainable development.

9.   Track II Diplomacy: Informal, non-governmental channels of diplomacy, known as Track II diplomacy, involve academics, experts, and civil society organizations. These actors can help facilitate dialogue and build trust between conflicting parties.

10.   Public Diplomacy: Governments use public diplomacy to engage with foreign publics and influence their perceptions. This can include cultural exchanges, educational programs, and media campaigns.

Challenges to International Cooperation

While international cooperation is vital, it is not without challenges. Here are some of the obstacles that can hinder effective collaboration among nations:

1.   National Interests: Nations often prioritize their own interests over global ones. This can lead to reluctance in cooperating on issues that may not align with a country's short-term goals.

2.   Political Differences: Ideological and political differences between nations can impede cooperation. For instance, tensions between democratic and authoritarian regimes can hinder consensus in international forums.

3.   Resource Allocation: Disputes over resource distribution, whether it's access to water, minerals, or energy sources, can strain international relations.

4.   Trust Deficits: Building trust among nations can be challenging, especially after conflicts or disagreements. Mutual suspicion can hinder cooperation efforts.

5.   Coordination Challenges: Coordinating actions among numerous countries with different agendas can be complex and time-consuming.

6.   Lack of Enforcement Mechanisms: Some international agreements lack effective enforcement mechanisms, making it difficult to hold nations accountable for violations.

7.   Nationalism and Populism: The rise of nationalist and populist movements in various countries can lead to a more inward-focused approach, making international cooperation less politically appealing.

8.   Technological Challenges: Emerging technologies, such as cyber warfare capabilities, can be used to disrupt international cooperation efforts.

Strategies to Enhance International Cooperation

Given these challenges, it's crucial to identify strategies that can enhance international cooperation:

1.   Diplomatic Engagement: Actively engaging in diplomatic efforts and negotiations can help build bridges between nations.

2.   Building Trust: Confidence-building measures and transparent communication can foster trust between countries.

3.   Conflict Resolution: Investing in effective conflict resolution mechanisms can prevent disputes from escalating and obstructing cooperation.

4.   Incentives: Offering incentives for cooperation, such as economic benefits or technology sharing, can motivate nations to work together.

5.   Global Governance Reform: Reforming international institutions to make them more inclusive, transparent, and effective can enhance cooperation.

6.   Public Awareness: Educating the public about the importance of international cooperation can generate support for global initiatives.

7.   Science and Technology Cooperation: Collaborative research and innovation projects can strengthen ties between nations and address global challenges.

8.   Track II Diplomacy: Informal dialogues and citizen diplomacy can complement official diplomatic efforts.

Case Studies in International Cooperation

To illustrate the principles and strategies of international cooperation, let's examine some notable case studies:

1.   The European Union: The EU is a prime example of regional cooperation. It has promoted peace, economic integration, and political stability among its member states. Through the single market and common currency (the Euro), the EU has achieved unprecedented economic cooperation.
2.   The Paris Agreement: The Paris Agreement, adopted in 2015, represents a landmark in global climate cooperation. Nations around the world committed to reducing greenhouse gas emissions to combat climate change. The agreement relies on a bottom-up approach, allowing countries to set their own targets, which enhances participation.
3.   The Marshall Plan: After World War II, the United States initiated the Marshall Plan to aid the reconstruction of Europe. This economic assistance not only helped rebuild war-torn nations but also fostered cooperation and stability in the region.
4.   The Joint Comprehensive Plan of Action (JCPOA): The JCPOA, also known as the Iran Nuclear Deal, was an agreement between Iran and major world powers aimed at limiting Iran's nuclear program in exchange for sanctions relief. While it faced challenges, it demonstrated that diplomatic solutions are possible even in complex geopolitical situations.
5.   The International Space Station (ISS): The ISS is a remarkable example of international cooperation in science and technology. It involves space agencies from multiple countries, including NASA (United States), Roscosmos (Russia), ESA (European Space Agency), JAXA (Japan Aerospace Exploration Agency), and CSA (Canadian Space Agency). These agencies collaborate on research, experiments, and the operation of the space station, showcasing how nations can work together beyond Earth's boundaries for mutual benefit.

6.   The United Nations Peacekeeping Operations: UN peacekeeping missions are critical for maintaining peace and security in conflict zones. Nations contribute troops and resources to these missions, illustrating a collective commitment to preventing and resolving conflicts.
7.   The World Trade Organization (WTO): The WTO plays a central role in regulating international trade and resolving trade disputes. Its rules-based system has helped reduce trade barriers and promote economic cooperation among member countries.
8.   The G20: The Group of Twenty (G20) is a forum for the world's major economies to discuss global economic issues. It showcases how leading nations can collaborate on financial stability, economic growth, and development.
9.   Humanitarian Response to Natural Disasters: When natural disasters strike, international cooperation is evident through the rapid deployment of humanitarian aid

and relief efforts. Organizations like the Red Cross and United Nations agencies coordinate assistance from various countries to provide relief to affected regions.

10.   Global Health Initiatives: Initiatives like GAVI (Global Alliance for Vaccines and Immunization) and the Global Fund to Fight AIDS, Tuberculosis, and Malaria demonstrate how countries and organizations collaborate to combat global health challenges.

Challenges in Recent International Cooperation Efforts

While these case studies highlight successful international cooperation, they also reveal ongoing challenges:

1.   The United Nations Security Council: The Security Council's structure, with its five permanent members wielding veto power, has been a source of frustration and ineffectiveness in addressing global conflicts. Reforms to make it more representative and accountable have been slow to materialize.

2.   The Refugee Crisis: The global refugee crisis, triggered by conflicts and persecution, has strained international cooperation. Nations have often struggled to share the responsibility of hosting and assisting refugees adequately.

3.   Trade Disputes: Trade tensions and disputes, such as those between the United States and China, have tested the effectiveness of multilateral trade organizations like the WTO. Finding common ground on trade policies remains a challenge.

4.   Climate Action: Despite international agreements like the Paris Agreement, achieving meaningful progress on climate change remains difficult. Some nations have been slow to implement their commitments, and climate negotiations often face political obstacles.

5.   Pandemic Response: The COVID-19 pandemic revealed gaps in international cooperation in responding to global health crises. Vaccine distribution, intellectual property rights, and equitable access to medical resources have been contentious issues.

International cooperation is the cornerstone of a peaceful, prosperous, and sustainable world. In an era marked by complex global challenges, ranging from climate change to global health crises, no nation can address these issues in isolation. Strategies like diplomacy, international agreements, and multilateral organizations provide the framework for nations to collaborate effectively.

However, challenges such as national interests, political differences, and a lack of trust can hinder cooperation. Overcoming these challenges requires diplomatic skill, transparent communication, and a commitment to finding common ground. The case studies mentioned demonstrate that international cooperation is not only possible but also essential for addressing the most pressing issues of our time.

As the world continues to evolve, it is imperative that nations, organizations, and individuals recognize the interdependence of our global community. By embracing the principles of international cooperation and pursuing strategies to enhance collaboration, we can build a better future for all. Whether it's through joint efforts in diplomacy, science, economics, or humanitarian aid, cooperation remains our most potent tool in shaping a more interconnected and harmonious world.

Vaccines and Therapeutics

The fields of vaccines and therapeutics have been pivotal in shaping the course of human health and medical progress throughout history. These two branches of medicine play distinct yet interconnected roles in preventing and treating diseases. Vaccines primarily focus on disease prevention by stimulating the body's immune system to produce a protective response against specific pathogens, while therapeutics involve the use of drugs and interventions to manage and treat existing diseases. In this comprehensive exploration, we will delve into the evolution of vaccines and therapeutics, their impact on public health, the challenges they face, and the future prospects of these crucial medical interventions.

I. Historical Evolution of Vaccines

Vaccination, a term derived from the Latin word "vacca" for cow, has a rich history that dates back centuries. The practice of inoculation and vaccination has been used in various forms to combat infectious diseases. One of the earliest examples is the smallpox inoculation technique, developed in Asia and Africa. Variolation, as it was known, involved the deliberate introduction of smallpox material into a person's skin, leading to a milder form of the disease and immunity.

1.   Edward Jenner and the Smallpox Vaccine
The development of the smallpox vaccine by Edward Jenner in 1796 is a milestone in the history of vaccines. Jenner observed that individuals who contracted cowpox, a less severe disease, seemed to be immune to smallpox. He conducted experiments by inoculating individuals with material from cowpox lesions, which led to immunity against smallpox. This breakthrough marked the birth of modern vaccination and laid the foundation for future vaccine development.
2.   The Vaccine Revolution
The success of the smallpox vaccine paved the way for the development of vaccines against other infectious diseases. Throughout the 19th and 20th centuries, vaccines for diseases such as rabies, polio, tetanus, and diphtheria were developed, drastically reducing the burden of these illnesses. The introduction of mass vaccination campaigns in the mid-20th century further accelerated the control and eradication of various diseases.

II. Impact of Vaccines on Public Health

Vaccines have had a profound impact on public health by preventing the spread of infectious diseases and reducing morbidity and mortality rates. Here are some key examples of how vaccines have shaped public health:

1.   Smallpox Eradication

The global smallpox eradication campaign, spearheaded by the World Health Organization (WHO) and carried out from 1967 to 1980, stands as one of the most significant achievements in public health history. Through widespread vaccination efforts, smallpox was successfully eradicated, marking the first and only time a human disease has been eradicated through vaccination.

2.   Polio and the Near Eradication Effort

Vaccination has also been instrumental in the near eradication of polio. The Global Polio Eradication Initiative, launched in 1988, has made substantial progress in reducing polio cases worldwide. This initiative relies heavily on oral polio vaccines, demonstrating the power of vaccines in controlling infectious diseases.

3.   The Decline of Vaccine-Preventable Diseases

Vaccines have contributed to a significant decline in the incidence of diseases such as measles, mumps, rubella, and pertussis (whooping cough). These vaccines have been integrated into routine childhood immunization programs, resulting in substantial reductions in disease prevalence.

III. Challenges in Vaccination

While vaccines have been instrumental in reducing the burden of infectious diseases, they face various challenges in their development, distribution, and acceptance.

1.   Vaccine Hesitancy

Vaccine hesitancy, fueled by misinformation and distrust, has become a global concern. Some individuals and communities are reluctant to receive vaccines due to fears of adverse effects or mistrust of the healthcare system. Addressing vaccine hesitancy requires effective communication and education.

2.   Vaccine Development and Approval

The process of developing and approving vaccines can be lengthy and resource-intensive. Ensuring vaccine safety and efficacy is crucial but can lead to delays, especially during outbreaks. Streamlining these processes without compromising safety is a continuous challenge.

3.   Access and Equity

Disparities in vaccine access exist both within and between countries. Low- and middle-income countries often struggle to procure and distribute vaccines, leading to unequal protection against diseases. Achieving equitable vaccine access remains a global goal.

IV. The Therapeutics Landscape

Therapeutics encompass a wide range of medical interventions designed to treat diseases, alleviate symptoms, and improve patients' quality of life. Therapeutic approaches have evolved significantly over time, influenced by scientific advancements and our growing understanding of diseases.

1.   Pharmaceutical Therapies
Pharmaceutical therapeutics, including drugs and biologics, play a central role in modern medicine. The development of antibiotics revolutionized the treatment of bacterial infections, while advancements in oncology have led to targeted therapies and immunotherapies for cancer.
2.   Surgical and Procedural Interventions
Surgical and procedural interventions are essential therapeutic options for conditions that cannot be managed solely with medication. Surgeries, such as organ transplantation, joint replacement, and minimally invasive procedures, have extended and improved the lives of countless patients.
3.   Gene and Cell Therapies
Recent breakthroughs in gene and cell therapies have opened new frontiers in therapeutics. These innovative approaches hold promise for treating genetic disorders, regenerating damaged tissues, and potentially curing previously incurable diseases.

V. The Intersection of Vaccines and Therapeutics

Vaccines and therapeutics are often seen as distinct approaches in medicine, but there is an increasing overlap between them, particularly in the field of immunotherapy. Here are some examples of this intersection:

1.   Cancer Immunotherapy
Cancer vaccines and immunotherapies, such as checkpoint inhibitors and CAR-T cell therapies, harness the immune system to target and destroy cancer cells. These therapies represent a convergence of vaccine principles with therapeutic goals.
2.   Therapeutic Vaccines
Some vaccines are designed not only to prevent disease but also to treat existing infections or conditions. Therapeutic vaccines aim to stimulate the immune system to combat diseases like HIV and certain types of cancer.
3.   Antibody Therapies
Monoclonal antibodies, derived from the principles of vaccination, are used as therapeutics to neutralize pathogens or treat autoimmune diseases. The development of monoclonal antibody therapies for COVID-19 highlighted their potential in managing infectious diseases.

VI. Challenges in Therapeutics

Therapeutics face their own set of challenges, some of which are shared with vaccines, while others are unique:

1.   Drug Resistance

The emergence of drug-resistant pathogens, including bacteria and viruses, poses a significant challenge to therapeutics. Antimicrobial resistance threatens our ability to treat infectious diseases effectively.

2.   High Costs

Many advanced therapeutics, especially gene and cell therapies, come with high costs. Ensuring affordability and equitable access to these treatments remains a major concern.

3.   Regulatory Hurdles

The approval and regulation of therapeutics involve complex processes that can delay patient access to innovative treatments. Streamlining regulatory pathways while maintaining safety standards is an ongoing challenge.

VII. Future Prospects and Innovations

The future of vaccines and therapeutics holds exciting possibilities driven by scientific advancements and technological breakthroughs:

1.   mRNA Vaccines and Therapies

The success of mRNA vaccines against COVID-19 has paved the way for their application in other vaccines and therapeutic areas, including cancer and infectious diseases.

AI-Driven Drug Discovery

Artificial intelligence (AI) and machine learning are transforming drug discovery and development. These technologies can analyze vast datasets to identify potential drug candidates, predict their efficacy, and accelerate the drug development process.

3.   Personalized Medicine

The era of personalized medicine is dawning, where treatments are tailored to an individual's genetic makeup and specific disease characteristics. This approach has the potential to optimize therapeutic outcomes and reduce side effects.

4.   CRISPR and Gene Editing

CRISPR-Cas9 and other gene-editing technologies offer the ability to modify the human genome, potentially providing cures for genetic diseases. These tools also hold promise in developing therapeutics for conditions like cancer and HIV.

5.   Immunotherapies Beyond Cancer

Immunotherapies, such as CAR-T cell therapies, are being explored for applications beyond cancer, including autoimmune diseases and infectious diseases. This expanding field could revolutionize the treatment of a wide range of conditions.

6.   Pandemic Preparedness

The COVID-19 pandemic highlighted the importance of rapid vaccine development and distribution. Efforts are underway to establish global systems for faster responses to emerging infectious diseases, improving pandemic preparedness.

VIII. Ethical and Societal Considerations

As vaccines and therapeutics continue to advance, it is essential to consider the ethical and societal implications associated with their development and deployment:

1.   Equity in Access

Ensuring equitable access to vaccines and therapeutics remains a moral imperative. Global efforts must be made to bridge the gap between developed and developing countries in terms of access to life-saving treatments.

2.   Informed Consent

Ethical concerns surrounding informed consent become crucial, especially in clinical trials and experimental therapies. Patients and participants must have a clear understanding of the risks and benefits associated with these interventions.

3.   Surveillance and Privacy

The collection of health data for vaccine distribution and monitoring may raise concerns about privacy and data security. Striking a balance between public health surveillance and individual privacy is an ongoing challenge.

4.   Vaccine Mandates and Policies

The implementation of vaccine mandates and policies can be contentious. Balancing public health goals with individual freedoms and rights requires careful consideration and public engagement.

Vaccines and therapeutics have been instrumental in improving human health and longevity throughout history. From the eradication of smallpox to the development of cutting-edge gene therapies, these medical interventions continue to shape the course of medicine and healthcare.

While both vaccines and therapeutics face unique challenges and ethical considerations, they also offer tremendous opportunities for innovation and progress. The intersection of these fields, especially in areas like immunotherapy, holds promise for novel treatments and cures.

As we look to the future, it is imperative that we prioritize equity in access, ethical principles, and scientific collaboration to ensure that vaccines and therapeutics continue to benefit all of humanity. The ongoing pursuit of scientific knowledge and the responsible application of medical advancements will be key in addressing the health challenges of tomorrow.

Managing Epidemics and Pandemics

Epidemics and pandemics have been recurring challenges throughout human history. From the Black Death in the 14th century to the more recent COVID-19 pandemic, these health crises have left indelible marks on societies worldwide. In this comprehensive exploration, we will delve into the multifaceted world of managing epidemics and pandemics, analyzing the key components of preparedness, response, and recovery.

I. Understanding Epidemics and Pandemics

To effectively manage epidemics and pandemics, we must first comprehend the terminology and characteristics that define them.

1.   Definition and Distinction:
•   Epidemic: An outbreak of a disease that occurs in a defined geographic area and affects an unusually large number of people.
•   Pandemic: A global epidemic that affects a substantial portion of the world's population, often caused by a new infectious agent.
2.   Characteristics:
•   Rapid Spread: Epidemics and pandemics can spread quickly due to globalization, travel, and urbanization.
•   Novel Pathogens: Many pandemics result from new or mutated pathogens that humans have limited immunity to.
•   Societal Impact: These events impact healthcare systems, economies, and daily life, often causing widespread disruption.

II. Preparedness

Effective preparedness is the cornerstone of managing epidemics and pandemics. This phase involves proactive measures aimed at reducing vulnerability and enhancing response capabilities.

1.   Surveillance and Early Detection:
•   Robust surveillance systems monitor disease trends, detect outbreaks early, and enable timely interventions.
•   Advanced technology, such as machine learning and data analytics, aids in predicting outbreaks.
2.   Risk Assessment and Contingency Planning:
•   Governments and organizations assess the potential impact of various pathogens and develop contingency plans.

•	These plans outline response strategies, resource allocation, and communication protocols.
3.	Healthcare Infrastructure:
•	Building and maintaining a resilient healthcare infrastructure is crucial.
•	Adequate healthcare facilities, medical supplies, and a skilled workforce are essential.
4.	Research and Development:
•	Investment in research accelerates vaccine and treatment development.
•	Platforms like mRNA vaccines have shown rapid response capabilities during pandemics.
5.	Public Health Education:
•	Public awareness campaigns promote hygiene, vaccination, and responsible behavior.
•	Prepared communities are more resilient during health crises.

III. Response

When an epidemic or pandemic occurs, a swift and well-coordinated response is imperative to mitigate the spread and minimize the impact.

1.	Incident Management:
•	Activation of emergency response teams and incident command centers ensures coordination.
•	Clear leadership and communication structures are critical.
2.	Healthcare Delivery:
•	Hospitals and healthcare providers play a pivotal role in treating patients and preventing further transmission.
•	Prioritizing resources and implementing surge capacity plans are essential.
3.	Vaccination and Treatment:
•	Mass vaccination campaigns are key in pandemic response.
•	Antiviral treatments and therapies reduce the severity of illness.
4.	Quarantine and Isolation:
•	Quarantine measures restrict movement to contain the spread.
•	Isolation separates infected individuals from others to prevent transmission.
5.	Communication:
•	Timely and accurate information dissemination builds trust and ensures compliance with public health measures.
•	Countering misinformation and rumors is vital.
6.	International Collaboration:
•	Global cooperation through organizations like the WHO facilitates information sharing and resource allocation.

- Collaborative research accelerates vaccine and treatment development.

IV. Recovery

After the immediate crisis, communities and nations must focus on recovery and resilience-building.

1. Healthcare System Strengthening:
- Post-pandemic, healthcare systems require reinforcement to handle ongoing healthcare needs.
- Investment in healthcare infrastructure and workforce is crucial.
2. Mental Health Support:
- Pandemics take a toll on mental health, necessitating comprehensive support services.
- Accessible counseling and mental health programs are essential.
3. Economic Recovery:
- Pandemics have severe economic consequences.
- Governments implement stimulus packages and support for affected industries.
4. Lessons Learned:
- Conducting post-pandemic evaluations identifies strengths and weaknesses.
- These lessons inform future preparedness efforts.

V. Case Studies

To gain practical insights into managing epidemics and pandemics, we can analyze notable historical and recent examples.

1. The Spanish Flu (1918):
- A devastating influenza pandemic.
- Limited medical knowledge and resources hampered response efforts.
- The importance of vaccination and healthcare infrastructure became apparent.
2. SARS (2002-2003):
- Severe Acute Respiratory Syndrome (SARS) led to a global outbreak.
- Swift international cooperation helped contain the virus.
- Enhanced surveillance and quarantine measures were implemented.
3. Ebola Outbreak (2014-2016):
- An outbreak in West Africa.
- Highlighted the importance of rapid response and international aid.
- Strengthened global preparedness for future outbreaks.
4. COVID-19 Pandemic (2019-ongoing):
- The most recent and ongoing global pandemic.

- Demonstrated the critical role of scientific innovation and vaccine distribution.
- Exposed vulnerabilities in healthcare systems and misinformation challenges.

VI. Challenges and Ethical Considerations

Managing epidemics and pandemics presents numerous challenges and ethical dilemmas.

1. Equity in Access:
- Ensuring equal access to vaccines and treatments across nations and socioeconomic groups is a challenge.
2. Misinformation:
- The rapid spread of misinformation can hinder public health efforts.
- Fact-checking and education are crucial.
3. Quarantine and Privacy:
- Balancing public health with individual privacy rights is an ongoing debate.
- Contact tracing apps and data privacy concerns arise.
4. Vaccine Hesitancy:
- Vaccine hesitancy undermines vaccination campaigns.
- Public education and addressing concerns are necessary.
5. Global Cooperation:
- Achieving international collaboration can be challenging due to political and economic interests.
- Stronger frameworks for cooperation are needed.

VII. Future Prospects

The world of epidemic and pandemic management is constantly evolving, with several promising developments on the horizon.

1. Vaccine Technology:
- Advancements in vaccine technology, like mRNA vaccines, offer rapid response capabilities.
2. AI and Data Analytics:
- Artificial intelligence and data analytics continue to enhance disease surveillance and prediction.
3. Global Health Security:
- Investment in global health security infrastructure is increasing.
- Initiatives like the Global Health Security Agenda aim to improve preparedness.
4. Pandemic Preparedness Agreements:

- International agreements and treaties may be established to streamline response efforts.
5.   One Health Approach:
- The One Health approach recognizes the interconnectedness of human, animal, and environmental health.
- It aims to prevent zoonotic diseases at their source.

Managing epidemics and pandemics is a complex, multifaceted challenge that demands global cooperation, preparedness, and resilience. The lessons learned from historical and contemporary outbreaks have provided valuable insights into response strategies and the importance of scientific innovation. As we continue to navigate an ever-changing landscape of infectious diseases, it is imperative that we remain vigilant, adaptable, and committed to protecting public health on a global scale.

Surveillance and Data Analysis

Epidemics and pandemics have been recurring challenges throughout human history. From the Black Death in the 14th century to the Spanish flu in the early 20th century, infectious diseases have had devastating impacts on societies. In recent times, the COVID-19 pandemic has once again highlighted the critical importance of surveillance and data analysis in understanding, managing, and mitigating the effects of such health crises.

This essay delves into the role of surveillance and data analysis in epidemics and pandemics. It explores how data collection, analysis, and dissemination have evolved over time, the ethical considerations surrounding these practices, and their implications for public health, privacy, and policymaking.

Section 1: Historical Context

1.1 The Role of Surveillance in Epidemics

Surveillance, in the context of epidemics, refers to the systematic monitoring of disease occurrence, spread, and impact within a population. Historically, surveillance was primarily conducted through direct observation and reports from healthcare professionals and the public. During the 19th and early 20th centuries, techniques such as quarantine and isolation were used to control the spread of diseases like cholera and tuberculosis.

1.2 Advancements in Data Collection

The 20th century saw significant advancements in data collection methods. The introduction of electronic health records, laboratory testing, and epidemiological surveys improved the accuracy and timeliness of data collection. However, data collection remained fragmented and often relied on manual reporting, leading to delays in response.

Section 2: Modern Surveillance and Data Analysis

2.1 The Digital Revolution

The digital revolution of the late 20th and early 21st centuries transformed the landscape of epidemic surveillance. The proliferation of the internet, mobile devices, and electronic health records allowed for the real-time collection and analysis of vast amounts of health-related data. This data includes information on symptoms, travel history, and contact tracing, which are crucial for tracking and controlling the spread of infectious diseases.

2.2 Data Integration and Analytics

Modern surveillance systems rely on data integration and advanced analytics. Machine learning algorithms, artificial intelligence, and predictive modeling have become indispensable tools for identifying disease outbreaks, assessing their potential impact, and devising effective response strategies. These technologies enable health authorities to detect anomalies and patterns in data that may indicate the emergence of a new disease or the resurgence of a known one.

2.3 The Role of Big Data

The concept of "big data" has gained prominence in the field of epidemiology. Big data analytics involve processing and analyzing vast and diverse datasets to extract meaningful insights. In the context of epidemics, big data can include social media posts, geolocation data from smartphones, and even satellite imagery to monitor population movement and predict disease spread.

2.4 Contact Tracing Apps

The COVID-19 pandemic highlighted the importance of contact tracing. Mobile applications that use Bluetooth technology to track interactions between individuals have been developed and deployed in many countries. These apps have faced challenges related to privacy concerns and adoption rates but have also demonstrated their potential to enhance traditional contact tracing methods.

Section 3: Ethical Considerations

3.1 Balancing Privacy and Public Health

One of the most significant ethical dilemmas in epidemic surveillance is the tension between individual privacy and public health. Collecting and sharing personal health data, especially in real-time, raises concerns about surveillance overreach and data security. Striking a balance between protecting public health and safeguarding individual rights is an ongoing challenge.

3.2 Informed Consent

The use of personal data for epidemic surveillance raises questions about informed consent. Individuals must be aware of how their data is collected, used, and shared. Obtaining explicit consent for data collection is crucial, but it can be challenging in emergencies when swift action is required.

3.3 Data Accuracy and Transparency

The accuracy of data used in epidemic surveillance is paramount. Misinformation and data errors can lead to ineffective responses and erode public trust. Maintaining transparency in data collection and analysis methods is essential to building and maintaining trust in surveillance efforts.

Section 4: Implications for Public Health

4.1 Early Detection and Rapid Response

Effective surveillance and data analysis enable early detection of outbreaks, which is crucial for a rapid response. Identifying cases, isolating individuals, and implementing public health measures promptly can prevent the exponential spread of infectious diseases.

4.2 Resource Allocation

Data analysis helps allocate resources efficiently. By understanding the geographic and demographic patterns of disease spread, health authorities can direct medical supplies, personnel, and testing facilities to where they are needed most.

4.3 Vaccine Distribution

Surveillance data plays a critical role in vaccine distribution. Identifying high-risk populations and monitoring vaccine coverage can ensure equitable access to vaccines and enhance community immunity.

Section 5: Policy and Governance

5.1 International Cooperation

Epidemics and pandemics are global challenges that require international cooperation. Organizations like the World Health Organization (WHO) coordinate surveillance efforts, data sharing, and response strategies among countries. Collaborative research and data exchange are essential for a coordinated global response.

5.2 Data Sharing and Standardization

The harmonization of data sharing standards is vital for effective surveillance. Different countries and regions may use varying data formats and definitions, hindering cross-border analysis. Standardization efforts aim to address these disparities and facilitate data exchange.

5.3 Legal Frameworks

Many countries have established legal frameworks for epidemic surveillance. These laws define the rights and responsibilities of individuals, healthcare providers, and government agencies regarding data collection, sharing, and use. Developing clear and ethical legal frameworks is an ongoing challenge, particularly in the context of emerging technologies.

Surveillance and data analysis are indispensable tools in the fight against epidemics and pandemics. As technology continues to advance, so too will our ability to monitor and respond to infectious diseases. However, ethical considerations, particularly regarding privacy and consent, must remain at the forefront of these efforts.

In an interconnected world, international cooperation and data sharing are essential for addressing global health threats. The lessons learned from the COVID-19 pandemic underscore the need for robust surveillance systems, transparent data practices, and agile policy responses.

While the future of epidemic surveillance will undoubtedly involve cutting-edge technologies, its success will ultimately depend on how well we navigate the ethical, legal, and social challenges inherent in collecting and analyzing data in the service of public health.

Public Health Interventions

Epidemics and pandemics have been recurring threats to humanity throughout history. From the Black Death in the 14th century to the Spanish flu in the 20th century, infectious diseases have had profound and far-reaching effects on societies worldwide. In recent years, the world has witnessed the devastating impact of the COVID-19 pandemic, which underscored the critical importance of effective public health interventions in controlling and mitigating the spread of infectious diseases. This essay explores the various public health interventions employed during epidemics and pandemics, their historical context, and their contemporary relevance in the context of the ongoing global health crisis.

I. Historical Perspective

Epidemics have shaped human history in profound ways. The impact of infectious diseases on societies, economies, and public health strategies has been a recurring theme throughout the centuries. Here, we examine some key historical epidemics and the public health interventions used to combat them.

A. The Black Death (1347-1351)

The Black Death, caused by the bacterium Yersinia pestis, was one of the deadliest pandemics in human history. It is estimated to have killed 75-200 million people across Europe, Asia, and Africa. During this time, public health interventions were rudimentary, with limited understanding of the disease's transmission.

1.   Quarantine: The concept of isolating those infected or potentially exposed to the disease began during the Black Death. Infected individuals and their households were often sealed off from the rest of the community to prevent further transmission.
2.   Personal Protection: People started using rudimentary protective gear, such as masks and clothing covering the entire body, to reduce the risk of infection.

B. The Spanish Flu (1918-1919)

The Spanish flu, caused by an H1N1 influenza virus, infected one-third of the world's population and resulted in an estimated 50 million deaths worldwide. Public health interventions during this pandemic included:

1.   Social Distancing: Measures such as closing schools, theaters, and public gatherings were implemented to reduce person-to-person transmission.

2.   Isolation and Quarantine: Infected individuals were isolated, and those exposed to the virus were quarantined.
3.   Hygiene and Masking: Public health campaigns emphasized the importance of hand hygiene and wearing masks.

II. Contemporary Public Health Interventions

Advancements in science and technology have revolutionized our ability to understand and combat epidemics and pandemics. Here, we explore modern public health interventions and their application in recent outbreaks, including the COVID-19 pandemic.

A. Disease Surveillance and Monitoring

1.   Epidemiological Surveillance: The systematic collection and analysis of data on disease occurrence and transmission are fundamental in identifying outbreaks early. Tools like electronic health records and real-time data sharing have improved surveillance capabilities.
2.   Contact Tracing: Utilizing digital tools and smartphone apps, contact tracing has become more efficient, allowing for rapid identification and isolation of potential cases.

B. Vaccination Programs

1.   Vaccine Development: Advances in molecular biology and vaccine technology have expedited the development of vaccines. The COVID-19 vaccines, developed in record time, highlight the potential of science in pandemic response.
2.   Mass Vaccination Campaigns: Governments and health organizations have implemented mass vaccination campaigns to achieve herd immunity and reduce the spread of the virus.

C. Pharmaceutical Interventions

1.   Antiviral Medications: Developing and distributing antiviral drugs, such as Remdesivir for COVID-19, can reduce the severity of the disease and its transmission.
2.   Therapeutic Treatments: Advancements in treatment protocols, such as the use of monoclonal antibodies, have improved patient outcomes.

D. Non-Pharmaceutical Interventions

1.   Social Distancing and Travel Restrictions: Implementing measures like lockdowns and travel restrictions can slow the spread of the virus.

2.   Mask Mandates: Wearing masks in public spaces has been widely adopted to reduce respiratory transmission.

E. Public Health Communication

1.   Risk Communication: Clear and consistent messaging from health authorities is essential in conveying information about the disease, preventive measures, and vaccination.
2.   Countering Misinformation: The spread of false information can hinder public health efforts. Governments and organizations have worked to combat misinformation through various channels.

III. Ethical Considerations

While public health interventions are crucial for containing epidemics and pandemics, ethical concerns often arise. Balancing public health with individual rights and liberties can be challenging. Here are some ethical considerations:

A. Privacy vs. Surveillance

The use of contact tracing apps and surveillance technology raises concerns about privacy infringement. Striking the right balance between public health surveillance and individual privacy is an ongoing debate.

B. Vaccine Mandates

Mandatory vaccination policies can spark debates about individual autonomy. Some argue that vaccines should be voluntary, while others believe that mandates are necessary to achieve herd immunity.

C. Access to Healthcare

Ensuring equitable access to vaccines and medical treatments is an ethical imperative. Disparities in healthcare access can exacerbate the impact of epidemics on vulnerable populations.

IV. Global Health and Cooperation

In an interconnected world, epidemics and pandemics are global challenges that require international cooperation. The COVID-19 pandemic highlighted the importance of coordinated responses and the need to address global health disparities.

A. International Collaboration

International organizations like the World Health Organization (WHO) play a central role in coordinating responses to global health crises. Collaboration among nations in sharing information and resources is vital.

B. Vaccine Equity

Efforts to distribute vaccines globally, such as COVAX, aim to ensure that low-income countries have equitable access to vaccines.

C. Preparedness

Investing in pandemic preparedness and response infrastructure is crucial. Lessons learned from past outbreaks can inform strategies for future epidemics.

V. Challenges and Lessons Learned

Despite advancements in public health interventions, challenges persist. The COVID-19 pandemic revealed several lessons for improving epidemic and pandemic management:

A. Global Supply Chains

Dependency on global supply chains for essential medical supplies and drugs can hinder response efforts. Building resilient supply chains is essential.

B. Communication

Effective risk communication and countering misinformation remain challenges. Public health agencies must continuously adapt their messaging strategies.

C. Vaccine Hesitancy

Vaccine hesitancy poses a significant obstacle to achieving herd immunity. Addressing concerns and promoting vaccine confidence are ongoing tasks.

Epidemics and pandemics have been part of human history, shaping societies and public health strategies. Throughout history, from the Black Death to the Spanish flu, public health interventions have evolved to combat these threats. In modern times, science and technology have transformed our ability to respond to outbreaks, as seen with the COVID-19 pandemic.

Ethical considerations, global cooperation, and ongoing challenges highlight the complexity of epidemic and pandemic management. As we look to the future, continued investment in public health infrastructure, research, and international collaboration will be key in ensuring a more effective response to these global health threats. The lessons learned from past pandemics underscore the importance of preparedness, communication, and equitable access to healthcare as we navigate the ever-evolving landscape of infectious diseases.

Part VI: Ethical, Legal, and Societal Considerations

Epidemics and pandemics have been recurring challenges throughout human history. These global health crises pose multifaceted challenges that extend beyond medical and scientific dimensions. Ethical, legal, and societal considerations play pivotal roles in shaping responses to such crises. In this discussion, we will delve into the intricate web of these considerations, exploring the ethical dilemmas, legal frameworks, and societal impacts associated with epidemics and pandemics.

I. Ethical Considerations

1. Allocation of Scarce Resources

One of the most pressing ethical dilemmas in epidemics and pandemics is the allocation of scarce resources, such as ventilators, vaccines, and hospital beds. The principle of distributive justice, which seeks to distribute resources fairly, is often put to the test. Decisions regarding who receives potentially life-saving treatment can be agonizing for healthcare professionals and policymakers.

2. Informed Consent and Privacy

Balancing public health interests with individual rights is another ethical challenge. The need for contact tracing and data collection to curb the spread of infectious diseases must be weighed against privacy concerns. Ensuring that individuals provide informed consent for testing and data sharing becomes crucial in this context.

3. Duty to Care vs. Personal Safety

Frontline healthcare workers face ethical dilemmas concerning their duty to care for patients and their own personal safety. The obligation to provide care during an epidemic can place immense physical and emotional burdens on these professionals. Ethical frameworks guide decision-making in these difficult situations.

4. Stigmatization and Discrimination

Epidemics often lead to the stigmatization of affected communities or individuals. Ethical considerations demand efforts to combat discrimination and promote empathy, understanding, and solidarity.

II. Legal Considerations

1. International Health Regulations

The World Health Organization (WHO) issues International Health Regulations that provide a legal framework for the management of international public health emergencies. These regulations define the rights and responsibilities of member states in responding to epidemics and pandemics, including notification, reporting, and collaboration.

2. Quarantine and Isolation Laws

Quarantine and isolation measures are essential tools in controlling the spread of infectious diseases. Legal frameworks must strike a balance between public health interests and individual liberties. Specific laws govern how, when, and for how long individuals can be quarantined or isolated.

3. Liability and Compensation

Legal considerations also extend to issues of liability and compensation. In cases where medical interventions or vaccines result in adverse effects, questions of responsibility and compensation for affected individuals or families arise. Establishing liability frameworks is essential.

4. Intellectual Property and Access to Medicines

During pandemics, there may be debates around intellectual property rights and access to essential medicines and vaccines. Legal mechanisms like compulsory licensing can be employed to ensure broader access to life-saving treatments.

III. Societal Considerations

1. Social Cohesion and Solidarity

Epidemics and pandemics test the strength of societies. Social cohesion and solidarity are crucial for successful responses. Communities that come together, support each other, and follow public health guidelines tend to fare better in managing the crisis.

2. Disparities and Vulnerable Populations

Societal considerations highlight the existing disparities in healthcare access and outcomes. Vulnerable populations, including low-income communities and racial minorities, are disproportionately affected by epidemics. Addressing these disparities becomes a societal imperative.

3. Mental Health Impacts

The mental health impacts of epidemics and pandemics are often underestimated. Isolation, fear, grief, and uncertainty take a toll on individuals and communities. Societal responses should prioritize mental health support.

4. Infodemic and Misinformation

The rapid spread of information, including misinformation, through digital channels has emerged as a societal challenge. Efforts to combat the "infodemic" become vital in ensuring accurate information reaches the public.

Epidemics and pandemics are complex challenges that transcend the realm of medicine and science. Ethical, legal, and societal considerations are integral components of the response to these crises. Striking a balance between public health imperatives, individual rights, and social well-being requires careful deliberation and collaboration. Effective management of these considerations is crucial to mitigating the impact of epidemics and pandemics on a global scale.

In conclusion, the ethical, legal, and societal dimensions of epidemics and pandemics form a tapestry of intricate challenges that society must navigate. By acknowledging and addressing these considerations, we can better prepare for and respond to future global health crises, ensuring a more equitable and compassionate world.

Ethical Dilemmas in Biowarfare

Biological warfare, often referred to as biowarfare, involves the use of biological agents, such as pathogens or toxins, to harm or kill individuals, animals, or plants. The development and potential use of bioweapons raise numerous ethical dilemmas, as the consequences of their deployment can be catastrophic. This article explores some of the key ethical issues surrounding biowarfare, including concerns about international law, human rights, the moral implications for scientists, and the role of governments in regulating bioweapons.

I. Historical Perspective

To understand the ethical dilemmas in biowarfare, it's essential to examine its historical context. The use of biological agents in warfare dates back centuries. In World War I, for instance, both the Allied and Central Powers explored the use of biological weapons. The horrors of these attempts led to the 1925 Geneva Protocol, which prohibited the use of biological and chemical weapons in warfare. However, ethical concerns remained, particularly during World War II and the Cold War, as nations continued researching bioweapons covertly.

II. International Laws and Treaties

One of the primary ethical dilemmas in biowarfare centers on international law and the enforcement of treaties. The Biological Weapons Convention (BWC) of 1972, which now has 183 member states, comprehensively bans the development, production, and possession of bioweapons. However, verifying compliance with the BWC is challenging, and there have been allegations of violations. The ethical question here is how to ensure adherence to these treaties and hold violators accountable while avoiding the risks of false accusations.

III. Human Rights and Biowarfare

Biological weapons have the potential to cause widespread suffering, death, and long-term health consequences. The use of bioweapons directly violates fundamental human rights, such as the right to life, health, and security. Ethical dilemmas arise when considering the balance between national security interests and the preservation of these rights. Governments must grapple with the question of whether the pursuit of bioweapons can ever be morally justifiable.

IV. Dual-Use Research

One ethical gray area in biowarfare is dual-use research, which involves scientific endeavors with both civilian and military applications. Research into infectious diseases, for example, can have both benevolent aims, such as vaccine development, and malevolent applications for bioweapon development. Scientists and institutions engaged in such research face ethical dilemmas concerning transparency, oversight, and the responsible sharing of information.

V. The Role of Scientists

Scientists play a critical role in biowarfare, as they are the ones who develop the knowledge and technologies behind bioweapons. Ethical concerns include questions about the responsibility of scientists to consider the potential harm caused by their work, the ethical oversight of their research, and the protection of scientific integrity. The Scientific Responsibility, Human Rights, and Law Program (SRHRL) has proposed guidelines to address these issues.

VI. Security and Oversight

Governments are tasked with ensuring the security of potentially dangerous biological agents and monitoring compliance with international treaties. Ethical dilemmas arise when determining the balance between national security interests and the need for transparency and oversight. Securing biowarfare research facilities and preventing unauthorized access to biological agents are paramount concerns.

VII. Emerging Biotechnologies

Advances in biotechnology, such as gene editing and synthetic biology, introduce new ethical dilemmas in biowarfare. These technologies can potentially enhance the virulence of pathogens or create entirely new bioweapons. The international community must grapple with regulating these emerging biotechnologies to prevent their misuse.

VIII. Crisis Management

In the event of a biowarfare attack or accidental release of a bioweapon, ethical considerations extend to crisis management. Governments must balance public safety, information transparency, and the need to avoid panic. The allocation of limited medical resources during a biological crisis also poses ethical challenges.

IX. Education and Awareness

To address ethical dilemmas in biowarfare effectively, there is a need for education and awareness among scientists, policymakers, and the general public. Ethical training and discussions about the responsible conduct of research in biotechnology fields are essential to foster a culture of biosecurity and ethics.

Ethical dilemmas in biowarfare are multifaceted and complex, spanning international law, human rights, scientific research, and government policies. Addressing these dilemmas requires a concerted effort from the global community, including governments, scientists, and ethical institutions. The principles of transparency, accountability, and the protection of human rights should guide efforts to prevent the development and use of bioweapons. Ultimately, the ethical imperative in biowarfare is to prioritize the well-being and safety of humanity while respecting the boundaries of science and international norms.

The Use of Biological Weapons

The use of biological weapons, often referred to as bioweapons or bioterrorism, has been a topic of concern and fascination for centuries. The deliberate use of biological agents to harm or kill humans, animals, or plants has the potential for catastrophic consequences. This essay aims to provide a comprehensive analysis of the use of biological weapons, examining their history, potential agents, effects, international efforts to control them, and the ethical and moral dilemmas surrounding their use.

I. Historical Perspective

The history of biological warfare dates back centuries. Early instances of using biological agents as weapons can be found in ancient texts and historical accounts. For example, in the 6th century B.C., the Assyrians reportedly contaminated their enemies' water supplies with the fungus rye ergot, causing symptoms of poisoning. Similarly, during the Middle Ages, besieging armies often used catapults to launch diseased animal carcasses into enemy fortifications to spread infectious agents. However, these early instances were rudimentary compared to the modern biological weapons we know today.

One of the most infamous episodes in the history of biological warfare occurred during World War II when Imperial Japan's Unit 731 conducted extensive experiments on humans, often resulting in their deaths, to develop biological weapons. The horrors of these experiments, including the dissemination of plague and anthrax, serve as a stark reminder of the potential for devastation associated with bioweapons.

II. Biological Agents

A wide range of biological agents can be used in bioweapons, including bacteria, viruses, fungi, and toxins. Some of the most concerning agents include:

1.   Anthrax: Bacillus anthracis, the bacterium responsible for anthrax, can form spores that are highly resistant and can survive in the environment for extended periods. Inhalation of anthrax spores can lead to severe respiratory distress and death.
2.   Smallpox: Variola virus, which causes smallpox, was declared eradicated in 1980. However, concerns remain about the virus's potential use as a bioweapon if it were to be reintroduced.
3.   Botulinum toxin: Produced by the bacterium Clostridium botulinum, this toxin is one of the most potent poisons known to humanity. It can cause paralysis and death when ingested or inhaled.

4.   Ebola virus: This highly lethal virus can cause severe hemorrhagic fever with a mortality rate of up to 90%. Its potential for use as a bioweapon raises significant concerns.
5.   Plague: Yersinia pestis, the bacterium responsible for plague, can be weaponized to cause outbreaks with high mortality rates.
6.   Influenza: Manipulating influenza viruses to enhance their virulence and transmissibility is a concern due to their potential to cause widespread pandemics.

III. Effects of Biological Weapons

The effects of biological weapons can vary widely depending on the agent used, the method of dissemination, and the population's vulnerability. Common consequences of bioweapon attacks include:

1.   High Mortality Rates: Many biological agents have the potential to cause widespread fatalities if not promptly controlled.
2.   Fear and Panic: Bioweapon attacks can instill fear and panic in affected populations, leading to social disruption and economic consequences.
3.   Long-term Health Effects: Survivors of bioweapon attacks may suffer from long-term health issues, including chronic illnesses and disabilities.
4.   Strain on Healthcare Systems: Bioweapon attacks can overwhelm healthcare systems, making it challenging to provide adequate care to the affected population.

IV. International Efforts to Control Biological Weapons

The international community has taken significant steps to control and prevent the use of biological weapons. One of the most crucial initiatives in this regard is the Biological Weapons Convention (BWC). Established in 1972, the BWC aims to prohibit the development, production, and acquisition of biological weapons and their delivery systems.

Key provisions of the BWC include:

1.   Prohibition: Signatory countries commit to never developing, producing, or using biological weapons.
2.   Verification: The treaty establishes a framework for verifying compliance with its provisions.
3.   Assistance and Cooperation: The BWC encourages international cooperation in preventing the misuse of biology for harmful purposes.
4.   Transparency: Member states are required to submit confidence-building measures and annual declarations regarding their biological research and activities.

Despite these efforts, challenges remain in verifying compliance and preventing the clandestine development of bioweapons. Advances in biotechnology and synthetic biology have further complicated the detection of potential violations.

V. Ethical and Moral Dilemmas

The use of biological weapons raises profound ethical and moral dilemmas. The intentional harm and suffering inflicted upon innocent civilians and combatants are clear violations of fundamental principles of human rights and humanitarian law. The indiscriminate nature of bioweapons, which can affect anyone within the path of exposure, amplifies these concerns.

Furthermore, the development and possession of biological weapons necessitate ethical considerations. Should scientists and researchers engage in the development of such weapons, even for defensive purposes? The potential dual-use nature of biotechnology compounds these ethical dilemmas, as technologies developed for legitimate research can be repurposed for harm.

VI. Contemporary Concerns and Emerging Threats

In the modern era, biological weapons pose new and evolving threats. Advances in biotechnology, including gene editing techniques like CRISPR-Cas9, have made it easier for individuals or groups with malicious intent to manipulate and potentially create dangerous biological agents. The global spread of information and expertise through the internet further heightens concerns about biosecurity.

Emerging threats include:

1.   Synthetic Biology: The ability to design and synthesize DNA has the potential to create entirely new biological agents or modify existing ones for nefarious purposes.
2.   Gene Editing: CRISPR technology can be used to enhance the virulence or resistance of pathogens, making them more lethal and harder to combat.
3.   Dual-Use Research: Scientific research with legitimate applications can be misused for harmful purposes, blurring the lines between defensive and offensive biotechnology.
4.   Global Connectivity: The interconnectedness of the modern world means that a bioweapon attack in one region can have far-reaching and global consequences.

VII. Preventing and Responding to Biological Weapons

Preventing the use of biological weapons requires a multifaceted approach:

1.   International Agreements: Strengthening and enforcing international agreements like the BWC is crucial to deter the use of bioweapons.
2.   Biosecurity Measures: Laboratories and research institutions must implement robust biosecurity measures to prevent unauthorized access to dangerous biological agents.
3.   Surveillance and Monitoring: Early detection and monitoring of disease outbreaks and suspicious activities are essential to identifying potential bioweapon threats.
4.   Education and Awareness: Public awareness campaigns can help inform the public about the risks of bioweapons and the importance of biosecurity.
5.   Response Preparedness: Governments must have well-developed response plans in case of bioweapon attacks, including the stockpiling of vaccines and treatments.

The use of biological weapons remains a grave concern in the contemporary world. While international efforts have been made to prohibit and control these weapons, emerging biotechnological advances create new challenges. Ethical considerations surrounding bioweapons persist, underscoring the need for responsible research and development practices.

Preventing and responding to biological weapons necessitate a collective global effort. Heightened vigilance, strong international agreements, and investment in biosecurity measures are essential to safeguarding humanity from the catastrophic consequences of bioweapon attacks.

Dual-Use Research and Ethics

In the realm of scientific research, there exists a unique and complex ethical dilemma known as "dual-use research." Dual-use research refers to scientific investigations and experiments that have the potential to yield both beneficial and harmful outcomes, with the potential for misuse or unintended consequences. This ethical challenge becomes particularly salient when considering research related to epidemics and pandemics, where the pursuit of knowledge to combat deadly diseases must be balanced against the risk of inadvertently creating new threats.

In this comprehensive exploration, we delve into the nuanced world of dual-use research and the ethical considerations it presents in the context of epidemic and pandemic research. We will discuss the definition of dual-use research, its historical context, its relevance to the fields of microbiology and virology, and the ethical frameworks that guide decision-making in this arena. Additionally, we will explore real-world examples of dual-use research in epidemics and pandemics and evaluate the measures in place to mitigate potential risks.

Defining Dual-Use Research

Before delving into the specifics of dual-use research in epidemics and pandemics, it is essential to establish a clear definition of what constitutes dual-use research. Dual-use research can be broadly defined as scientific research that has the potential for both beneficial and harmful applications, with the potential for misuse or unintended negative consequences. This duality arises from the dual nature of scientific knowledge, which can be harnessed for constructive purposes or exploited for destructive ends.

Historical Context

The concept of dual-use research is not new and can be traced back to the early days of science and technology. Throughout history, scientific discoveries and innovations have often been accompanied by ethical dilemmas related to their dual-use potential. For example, the discovery of nuclear fission in the 20th century brought about the development of both nuclear energy for peaceful purposes and nuclear weapons for destructive purposes.

In the context of epidemics and pandemics, dual-use research has been a recurring concern for several decades. The study of infectious diseases, particularly those caused by pathogens like bacteria and viruses, inherently carries the potential for dual-use. Researchers in microbiology and virology must grapple with the fact that their work can lead to advances in medical treatments and vaccine development, but it can also provide insights into the creation of bioweapons or the accidental release of dangerous pathogens.

Ethical Frameworks in Dual-Use Research

Ethical considerations play a pivotal role in guiding the conduct of dual-use research in the context of epidemics and pandemics. Several ethical frameworks and principles are relevant in this domain, including:

1.   The Precautionary Principle: This principle emphasizes the importance of taking preventive measures when scientific research has the potential for harm, even if the full extent of the risks is uncertain. In the context of dual-use research, the precautionary principle encourages researchers to consider the potential consequences of their work and take measures to minimize risks.
2.   The Dual-Use Dilemma: This ethical concept acknowledges the inherent tension between advancing scientific knowledge and protecting against potential harm. Researchers and institutions must strike a balance between promoting scientific progress and ensuring responsible conduct.
3.   Responsible Conduct of Research (RCR): RCR encompasses a set of ethical principles and guidelines that researchers should adhere to in their work. This includes transparency, integrity, and accountability in all aspects of research, especially when dealing with dual-use potential.
4.   Global Governance and Oversight: In the international context, organizations like the World Health Organization (WHO) and the Biological Weapons Convention (BWC) provide frameworks for governing and overseeing research with dual-use implications. These bodies aim to establish norms and standards to mitigate risks associated with such research.

Real-World Examples of Dual-Use Research

To better understand the practical implications of dual-use research in epidemics and pandemics, let's explore some real-world examples:

1.   Gain-of-Function Research: Gain-of-function (GoF) research involves manipulating pathogens to increase their transmissibility or virulence in a laboratory setting. While this research can provide valuable insights into how pathogens evolve and spread, it also raises concerns about the potential release of dangerous strains and the misuse of this knowledge.
2.   The 1918 Influenza Virus: In 2005, scientists successfully reconstructed the 1918 influenza virus, which caused a devastating pandemic. This research offered crucial

insights into the virus's virulence factors. However, it also raised ethical questions about the potential release of the reconstructed virus and its dual-use nature.

3.   The H5N1 Controversy: In 2011, researchers created a highly pathogenic H5N1 avian influenza strain that could potentially transmit between mammals. This research sparked a debate about whether the benefits of understanding the virus's mechanisms outweighed the risks associated with its creation.

Mitigating Risks and Ethical Considerations

The dual-use nature of research related to epidemics and pandemics presents a significant challenge for scientists, policymakers, and society as a whole. To mitigate the risks and uphold ethical standards, several strategies and considerations must be taken into account:

1.   Risk Assessment: Researchers must conduct thorough risk assessments before embarking on dual-use research. This includes evaluating the potential for harm, the likelihood of misuse, and the measures in place to prevent accidents or deliberate misuse.

2.   Biosafety and Biosecurity: Implementing stringent biosafety and biosecurity measures in laboratories is essential to prevent accidental releases of dangerous pathogens and unauthorized access to sensitive research.

3.   Ethical Oversight: Independent ethical review boards should assess research proposals with dual-use potential. These boards can provide recommendations and ensure that research is conducted responsibly and ethically.

4.   Dual-Use Education: Researchers and students in relevant fields should receive training and education on the ethical and safety considerations of dual-use research. This promotes awareness and responsible conduct.

5.   International Collaboration: Given the global nature of epidemics and pandemics, international cooperation and information sharing are crucial. Multilateral agreements and organizations can facilitate responsible research practices.

6.   Transparency and Reporting: Researchers should be transparent about their methods, findings, and any potential dual-use implications. Timely reporting of research outcomes helps the scientific community and policymakers assess risks.

7.   Public Engagement: Involving the public in discussions about dual-use research is essential for democratic decision-making. Public input can inform policy decisions and ensure that ethical considerations are addressed.

Dual-use research in the context of epidemics and pandemics represents a complex ethical challenge that demands careful consideration. Balancing the pursuit of scientific knowledge with the potential for harm or misuse is no easy task. However, by adhering to ethical principles, implementing rigorous safety measures, and fostering international collaboration, it is possible to navigate this terrain responsibly.

As the world continues to grapple with infectious diseases, the importance of dual-use research in advancing our understanding and response cannot be understated. Still, the ethical foundations that underpin this research must remain strong to safeguard against unintended consequences and promote the greater good of humanity. It is through responsible conduct and vigilant oversight that we can navigate the dual-use dilemma and harness the power of science to combat epidemics and pandemics while minimizing the risks they pose.

Legal Frameworks and Biowarfare

The world has witnessed unprecedented advancements in the field of biotechnology in recent decades. While these advancements have brought about remarkable benefits for medicine, agriculture, and various other sectors, they have also raised significant concerns about the potential misuse of biotechnology for malicious purposes, particularly in the form of biowarfare. Biowarfare, the use of biological agents to cause harm or death in humans, animals, or plants, poses a grave threat to global security and human existence. To address this threat, an intricate web of legal frameworks has been established at both national and international levels. This essay delves into the legal frameworks that govern biowarfare, explores their effectiveness, and highlights the evolving challenges presented by biotechnology in the realm of biological weapons.

I. Historical Context: From Antiquity to Modern Biowarfare

Biological warfare has a dark and enduring history that dates back to antiquity. Ancient civilizations, including the Romans, Greeks, and Persians, used primitive forms of biological weapons such as poisoned arrows and contaminated water supplies. However, it was not until the 20th century that the use of modern biowarfare agents became a significant concern.

1.   World War I: Early Concerns
During World War I, various countries explored the use of biological agents, including bacteria and toxins, as weapons. The most notable example was Germany's secret program to develop anthrax and glanders as biological weapons. The horrors of chemical warfare during this period led to the 1925 Geneva Protocol, which prohibited the use of bacteriological methods of warfare. However, the Protocol did not explicitly ban the development, production, or possession of biological weapons.
2.   World War II: The Dawn of Biowarfare
World War II saw the intensification of biowarfare research, particularly by the Japanese Imperial Army's notorious Unit 731. This unit conducted horrific experiments on humans and launched biological attacks on Chinese villages. Meanwhile, the Allies also researched biological weapons, albeit on a smaller scale. These wartime activities prompted growing international concern and laid the groundwork for post-war efforts to control biowarfare.

II. The Biological Weapons Convention (BWC): A Milestone in Legal Frameworks

The Biological Weapons Convention, also known as the BWC, stands as a cornerstone in the legal framework against biowarfare. Opened for signature in 1972 and entering into force in 1975, the BWC is an international treaty that prohibits the development, production, and acquisition of biological weapons. Its primary objectives include promoting peaceful uses of biological science and technology and preventing the use of biological agents for hostile purposes.

1.   Key Provisions of the BWC
a. Prohibition: The BWC categorically bans the development, production, and acquisition of biological weapons.
b. Verification: Parties to the BWC are obligated to provide information and cooperate in investigations to ensure compliance.
c. Assistance and Cooperation: The treaty encourages international cooperation for peaceful purposes while prohibiting assistance in biowarfare activities.
d. Destruction of Stockpiles: Parties possessing biological weapons are required to destroy them and related facilities.
2.   Challenges and Shortcomings
While the BWC represents significant progress in combating biowarfare, it has faced several challenges and shortcomings:
a. Lack of Verification Mechanisms: The BWC lacks robust verification mechanisms, making it difficult to detect non-compliance.
b. Ambiguity: The treaty's language can be vague and open to interpretation, complicating enforcement.
c. Advances in Biotechnology: Rapid advancements in biotechnology have raised concerns about the ease of covert bioweapons development.
d. Compliance Issues: Suspected violations of the BWC have occurred, such as the Soviet Union's biowarfare program during the Cold War.

III. National Legal Frameworks: Implementing BWC Obligations

To give effect to the BWC's provisions, countries have established national legal frameworks and regulatory mechanisms. These frameworks typically include legislation, regulations, and agencies responsible for enforcing compliance with the treaty.

1.   United States
The United States, as a party to the BWC, enacted the "Biological Weapons Anti-Terrorism Act of 1989." This act criminalizes the development, production, and acquisition of biological weapons, imposes penalties for violations, and establishes oversight by the Department of Justice and the Federal Bureau of Investigation.
2.   United Kingdom
The UK's Biological Weapons Act 1974 prohibits the development, possession, and use of biological weapons. Violations of this act are subject to severe penalties, including imprisonment.
3.   Russia

Russia, as a successor state to the Soviet Union, maintains a complex legal framework governing biological weapons. It has various laws and regulations aimed at preventing the proliferation of bioweapons materials and expertise.

These national legal frameworks play a crucial role in implementing the obligations of the BWC and serve as a deterrent against biowarfare activities within the respective countries. However, they are only effective if they are enforced rigorously and transparently.

IV. Evolving Threats: Biotechnology and Biowarfare

The landscape of biowarfare has evolved dramatically since the inception of the BWC. Recent advancements in biotechnology, genetic engineering, and synthetic biology have raised new challenges and concerns regarding the potential misuse of these technologies for biowarfare purposes.

1.   Dual-Use Dilemma
One of the primary challenges posed by biotechnology is the dual-use dilemma. Many scientific advancements and tools can be used for both peaceful and harmful purposes. For example, gene-editing technologies like CRISPR-Cas9, initially developed for medical and agricultural applications, can potentially be used to modify pathogens for biowarfare.

2.   Accessibility
The increasing accessibility of biotechnology tools and knowledge has lowered the barrier for individuals and non-state actors to engage in biowarfare-related activities. DIY biohacking communities and underground forums pose a potential risk for biowarfare proliferation.

3.   Rapid Bioweapon Development
Advancements in genetic engineering enable the rapid development of designer pathogens with enhanced virulence, drug resistance, or stealth capabilities. These could be used to create bioweapons with devastating effects.

4.   Attribution Challenges
Identifying the source of a biowarfare attack can be extremely challenging, especially when sophisticated techniques are used to conceal the origin. This raises questions about how to attribute responsibility and respond effectively.

V. International Efforts Beyond the BWC

Recognizing the evolving nature of biowarfare threats, international efforts have expanded beyond the BWC to address the challenges posed by biotechnology and emerging technologies.

1.   United Nations Security Council Resolution 1540
Adopted in 2004, UNSC Resolution 1540 imposes binding obligations on all UN member states to prevent the proliferation of nuclear, chemical, and biological weapons. It emphasizes the importance of securing biological materials and technologies.
2.   The Australia Group
This informal forum of countries aims to coordinate export controls to prevent the proliferation of chemical and biological weapons-related materials and technologies. It plays a crucial role in regulating the transfer of dual-use biotechnology items.
3.   The Global Health Security Agenda (GHSA)
GHSA is a multilateral initiative that focuses on strengthening global health security, including preparedness for biosecurity threats. It promotes collaboration among countries to enhance surveillance, detection, and response to infectious disease outbreaks.

VI. The Role of Non-Governmental Organizations (NGOs)

Non-governmental organizations (NGOs) play a pivotal role in complementing and monitoring the efforts of governments and international organizations in the realm of biowarfare prevention. These organizations often serve as watchdogs, advocates, and educators in the field of biosecurity.

1.   The Nuclear Threat Initiative (NTI)
NTI is a prominent NGO that focuses on reducing the risks associated with weapons of mass destruction, including biological weapons. NTI works to strengthen global biosecurity by fostering international collaboration, advocating for improved regulations, and raising awareness about the dangers of biowarfare.
2.   The International Federation of Biosafety Associations (IFBA)
IFBA is an organization dedicated to promoting biosafety and biosecurity worldwide. It provides training, guidance, and resources to enhance laboratory safety and security, reducing the risk of accidental releases or malicious use of dangerous pathogens.
3.   The Center for Biosecurity and Global Health
Based at the University of Nebraska Medical Center, this center conducts research, education, and policy analysis related to biosecurity and bioterrorism. It offers valuable insights into the evolving threats of biowarfare and strategies for mitigation.
4.   The Biosecurity Working Group
This group is a collaboration of experts from various fields who work to assess the risks posed by biotechnology and biowarfare. They publish reports, policy recommendations, and guidance on biosecurity issues.

VII. Challenges and Future Directions

While significant progress has been made in developing legal frameworks and international efforts to combat biowarfare, numerous challenges and uncertainties persist.

1. Compliance and Enforcement
Ensuring compliance with existing treaties and regulations remains a challenge, especially in the absence of robust verification mechanisms. The international community must strengthen measures to detect and penalize violators effectively.

2. Rapid Advancements in Biotechnology
Continued advancements in biotechnology, including gene editing, synthetic biology, and bioinformatics, make it increasingly difficult to anticipate and prevent biowarfare threats. Ongoing research is crucial to understanding and mitigating these risks.

3. Attribution and Accountability
Determining the source of a biowarfare attack is complex and may require significant time and resources. Developing better attribution methods and establishing accountability mechanisms for biowarfare incidents are essential.

4. Education and Public Awareness
Raising awareness about the dangers of biowarfare and the importance of biosecurity is vital. Education and outreach efforts must target both the scientific community and the general public to foster responsible conduct and reporting of suspicious activities.

5. International Cooperation
Enhancing international cooperation is essential in addressing biowarfare threats. Countries must collaborate on sharing information, technologies, and best practices to strengthen biosecurity globally.

6. Biosecurity Governance
The governance of biotechnology and biosecurity requires continuous adaptation to new challenges. International bodies and organizations must remain flexible and responsive to emerging threats.

The global community faces an ever-evolving threat in the form of biowarfare. While the Biological Weapons Convention represents a critical milestone in efforts to prevent biowarfare, the challenges posed by rapid advancements in biotechnology and the dual-use dilemma require ongoing attention and adaptation of legal frameworks.

National legal frameworks, international treaties, and the work of non-governmental organizations collectively contribute to biosecurity. However, achieving effective biosecurity demands not only legal and regulatory measures but also education, international cooperation, and vigilance.

The path forward involves strengthening existing legal frameworks, enhancing compliance and enforcement mechanisms, and embracing a culture of responsibility among scientists, policymakers, and the public. In an age where the potential consequences of biowarfare are more catastrophic than ever, the global community must unite to protect humanity from this perilous threat.

International Laws and Conventions

Epidemics and pandemics have been recurring challenges throughout human history, with diseases like the Black Death in the 14th century, the Spanish flu in the 20th century, and most recently, the COVID-19 pandemic in the 21st century, causing widespread devastation and loss of life. In response to these global health crises, international laws and conventions have been established to guide and govern the management and containment of epidemics and pandemics. This comprehensive exploration delves into the evolution of international laws and conventions on epidemic and pandemic management, their key provisions, their successes, and their limitations.

1.   Historical Context

The notion of international cooperation in dealing with epidemics and pandemics can be traced back to the 19th century when advances in transportation and trade made it evident that diseases could rapidly cross borders. One of the earliest international agreements related to public health was the International Sanitary Conferences held in the mid-19th century, which laid the foundation for future efforts in global health governance.

2.   The World Health Organization (WHO)

One of the most prominent organizations in global health governance is the World Health Organization (WHO), established in 1948 as a specialized agency of the United Nations (UN). The WHO plays a central role in coordinating international responses to epidemics and pandemics. Its constitution outlines its primary functions, including the collection of information on epidemics and the establishment of international health regulations (IHR).

3.   International Health Regulations (IHR)

The International Health Regulations (IHR) are a cornerstone of international law in the context of epidemic and pandemic management. First adopted in 1969 and later revised in 2005, the IHR provide a legal framework for countries to prevent the international spread of diseases while avoiding unnecessary interference with international traffic and trade. Key components of the IHR include the reporting of public health events, the establishment of national focal points, and the issuance of temporary recommendations by the WHO.

4.   The Role of the United Nations

The United Nations (UN) also plays a crucial role in addressing global health crises. The UN General Assembly has convened special sessions to discuss pandemics, and the United Nations Security Council has recognized the impact of diseases on international peace and security. This recognition has led to the inclusion of health concerns in broader peace and security discussions.

5.   Bilateral and Regional Agreements

In addition to international agreements, many countries have established bilateral and regional agreements related to epidemic and pandemic management. These agreements often facilitate the sharing of resources, expertise, and information during health emergencies. For example, the European Union has a dedicated agency, the European Centre for Disease Prevention and Control (ECDC), to coordinate responses to health threats.

6.   Successes and Challenges

Over the years, international laws and conventions have achieved notable successes in epidemic and pandemic management. For instance, the rapid containment of the 2014-2016 Ebola outbreak in West Africa was partly attributed to the implementation of the IHR. However, several challenges persist.

6.1 Successes

6.1.1. Smallpox Eradication

One of the most remarkable achievements in global health was the eradication of smallpox. This success was largely attributed to the concerted efforts of nations working under the guidance of the WHO. In 1980, the WHO officially declared smallpox eradicated, marking a significant milestone in the history of epidemic control.

6.1.2. Polio Eradication

Efforts to eradicate polio have also seen substantial progress, with only a few countries still reporting cases as of 2021. The Global Polio Eradication Initiative, launched in 1988, involves multiple international partners working together to eliminate the disease.

6.1.3. Response to COVID-19

The COVID-19 pandemic highlighted the importance of international cooperation in pandemic response. Despite challenges and criticisms, organizations like the WHO played a central role in coordinating global efforts to combat the virus. International collaboration led to the rapid development and distribution of vaccines, demonstrating the potential for collective action.

6.2 Challenges

6.2.1. Limited Enforcement Mechanisms

One of the main challenges in international epidemic and pandemic management is the lack of robust enforcement mechanisms. International laws and conventions often rely on voluntary compliance by member states, making it difficult to hold countries accountable for non-compliance.

6.2.2. Inequitable Access to Resources

During pandemics, there is often a glaring disparity in access to resources, including vaccines, diagnostics, and medical supplies. This inequity highlights the shortcomings of international agreements in ensuring equitable distribution and access, as wealthier nations tend to secure a disproportionate share of these resources.

6.2.3. Political Factors

Political considerations sometimes hinder effective international cooperation during pandemics. National interests and rivalries can lead to delays in sharing information, resources, and technologies, which can exacerbate the spread of diseases.

6.2.4. Challenges in Implementing IHR

While the IHR provides a robust framework for epidemic and pandemic management, not all countries have the capacity or resources to fully implement its provisions. Developing and least-developed nations may struggle to meet the IHR requirements, creating gaps in global health security.

7.   Recent Developments

The COVID-19 pandemic has prompted discussions on the need for reform and strengthening of the international legal framework for epidemic and pandemic management. Some key developments include:

7.1. COVAX Initiative

COVAX, led by Gavi, the Vaccine Alliance, the WHO, and the Coalition for Epidemic Preparedness Innovations (CEPI), aims to provide equitable access to COVID-19 vaccines worldwide. While COVAX has faced challenges in securing adequate vaccine supplies, it underscores the importance of global collaboration in pandemic response.

7.2. Proposed Pandemic Treaty

In 2021, a proposal for a new international pandemic treaty was put forward by several countries and organizations. This treaty, similar to the Framework Convention on Tobacco Control, seeks to enhance global preparedness and response to pandemics by strengthening international cooperation and coordination.

7.3. Discussions on Intellectual Property

The issue of intellectual property rights, particularly related to vaccines and treatments for COVID-19, has been a topic of intense debate. Some argue for temporary waivers on intellectual property rights to increase vaccine production and distribution, highlighting the tension between intellectual property and public health in the context of pandemics.

8.   Future Prospects

The ongoing challenges and lessons learned from past and current pandemics offer important insights into the future of international laws and conventions on epidemic and pandemic management.

8.1. Strengthening Enforcement Mechanisms

One avenue for improvement is the development of stronger enforcement mechanisms within international agreements. This could involve clearer consequences for non-compliance and mechanisms for dispute resolution.

8.2. Addressing Inequity

Efforts to address global health inequities should be a central focus. This includes measures to ensure equitable access to vaccines, treatments, and diagnostics, as well as capacity-building support for developing countries to better implement international health regulations.

8.3. Preparedness and Response

Enhancing global preparedness for pandemics is essential. This involves improving early warning systems, increasing stockpiles of medical supplies, and establishing rapid response teams that can be deployed to hotspots of emerging diseases.

8.4. Research and Innovation

Promoting research and innovation in the field of vaccines and treatments for emerging diseases should remain a priority. Encouraging collaboration between public and private sectors can accelerate the development and distribution of life-saving interventions.

International laws and conventions on epidemic and pandemic management have evolved over time, reflecting the global community's growing awareness of the need for collective action in the face of health crises. While these agreements have achieved significant successes, they also face persistent challenges, including enforcement issues, resource disparities, and political considerations.

The COVID-19 pandemic has underscored the importance of international cooperation in pandemic response and prompted discussions on reforms and new initiatives. Strengthening enforcement mechanisms, addressing global health inequities, enhancing preparedness, and promoting research and innovation are key areas for future development.

As the world continues to grapple with the complex and evolving nature of infectious diseases, the effectiveness of international laws and conventions will depend on the commitment of nations to work together, share resources, and prioritize the health and well-being of all people, regardless of their nationality or socioeconomic status. In an increasingly interconnected world, the management of epidemics and pandemics remains a collective responsibility that transcends borders and requires a unified global effort.

Prosecuting Biowarfare Crimes

Biological warfare, often referred to as biowarfare, represents one of the most insidious threats to humanity. The use of biological agents in warfare has the potential to cause widespread devastation, death, and long-term environmental and health consequences. As the world becomes increasingly interconnected, the need to address and prosecute biowarfare crimes becomes paramount. This comprehensive examination delves into the legal and ethical dimensions of prosecuting biowarfare crimes, the challenges faced in doing so, and potential strategies to strengthen the international community's response to this grave threat.

1.   Historical Context

Biological warfare is not a new concept. Throughout history, various cultures and societies have attempted to use pathogens and toxins as weapons. One notable example is the use of smallpox-infected blankets during the French and Indian War in the 18th century. However, the modern understanding of biowarfare emerged during the 20th century, with the development of advanced scientific knowledge and technologies.

The horrors of World War I saw the first widespread use of chemical agents, and concerns about biological warfare followed soon after. The Geneva Protocol of 1925, though primarily addressing chemical weapons, marked the first international agreement aimed at prohibiting the use of biological agents in warfare. Unfortunately, this prohibition did not deter certain nations from conducting research and stockpiling biowarfare agents during the following decades.

2.   Legal Framework

The legal framework governing biowarfare crimes consists of several key components:

2.1. The Biological Weapons Convention (BWC)

The Biological Weapons Convention, signed in 1972, is the cornerstone of international efforts to prohibit biological weapons. This treaty bans the development, production, acquisition, and stockpiling of biological weapons. It also requires the destruction of existing biological weapon stockpiles and encourages international cooperation in preventing the spread of biowarfare knowledge and materials. While the BWC is a crucial instrument, it lacks a robust verification mechanism, making enforcement challenging.

2.2. The Chemical Weapons Convention (CWC)

While primarily focused on chemical weapons, the Chemical Weapons Convention contains some provisions related to biowarfare. States parties to the CWC are obligated to declare any facilities that produce or process toxins and establish measures to control such facilities.

2.3. Customary International Law

Customary international law, including the Geneva Conventions, also plays a role in regulating biowarfare. These principles establish the protection of civilians and combatants from the use of biological agents in armed conflicts.

3.   Challenges in Prosecuting Biowarfare Crimes

Prosecuting biowarfare crimes presents numerous challenges:

3.1. Attribution

One of the most significant challenges is attributing a biowarfare attack to a specific entity or nation. Unlike conventional weapons, biological agents can be difficult to trace back to their source, as they can occur naturally. This ambiguity makes it challenging to hold responsible parties accountable.

3.2. Lack of Evidence

Gathering evidence to support prosecution can be exceptionally challenging in biowarfare cases. Often, these attacks leave behind limited physical evidence, making it difficult to build a strong case. Additionally, nations engaged in biowarfare may go to great lengths to conceal their activities.

3.3. Technical Expertise

Effectively prosecuting biowarfare crimes requires a deep understanding of biology, microbiology, and related fields. This necessitates collaboration between legal and scientific experts, which can be logistically complex and time-consuming.

3.4. International Cooperation

Biowarfare knows no borders, and the international community must cooperate to address this threat effectively. However, geopolitical tensions and mistrust can hinder such cooperation, making it difficult to establish a united front against biowarfare crimes.

4.   Recent Cases and Challenges

Several notable cases highlight the challenges and complexities of prosecuting biowarfare crimes:

4.1. The Aum Shinrikyo Cult

The Aum Shinrikyo cult's 1995 Tokyo subway sarin gas attack demonstrated the potential for non-state actors to use biological or chemical agents as weapons. While not a biowarfare incident in the traditional sense, this attack raised concerns about the ease with which a determined group could acquire and deploy such agents.

4.2. The Amerithrax Attacks

In 2001, a series of anthrax-laden letters were sent through the U.S. postal system, resulting in multiple deaths and infections. The investigation and prosecution of this case revealed the complexity of tracing the source of biological agents and the challenges in securing convictions.

4.3. The COVID-19 Pandemic

The COVID-19 pandemic, which began in late 2019, raised questions about the potential origins of the virus. While most experts believe it originated from natural sources, the possibility of a laboratory escape or intentional release has been the subject of speculation and investigation. This case underscores the difficulties in determining the true source of a biowarfare agent.

5.   Strengthening Prosecution Efforts

To address the challenges in prosecuting biowarfare crimes effectively, several strategies should be considered:

5.1. Strengthening the Biological Weapons Convention (BWC)

The BWC should be strengthened to include more robust verification measures. Enhanced transparency and information-sharing among member states can help detect and prevent biowarfare activities. This may involve more comprehensive reporting requirements and on-site inspections of facilities suspected of engaging in prohibited activities.

5.2. Improving International Cooperation

Enhanced international cooperation is essential for addressing biowarfare threats. Nations must work together to share information, intelligence, and expertise related to biological threats. This cooperation can be facilitated through international organizations like the United Nations and the World Health Organization (WHO).

5.3. Promoting Scientific Collaboration

Closer collaboration between the scientific and legal communities is crucial. Scientists can provide valuable expertise in identifying and characterizing biological agents, while legal experts can guide investigations and prosecutions. Initiatives that foster interdisciplinary collaboration can improve the ability to respond to biowarfare threats effectively.

5.4. Strengthening Domestic Legislation

Individual nations should enact and enforce robust domestic legislation that criminalizes biowarfare-related activities. This includes the possession, production, and dissemination of biological weapons and materials. Strong legal frameworks serve as a deterrent and provide the basis for prosecution when necessary.

5.5. Public Awareness and Education

Raising public awareness about the dangers of biowarfare and the importance of preventing it can help build support for stronger legal measures and international cooperation. Educational programs can inform citizens about the risks and consequences of biowarfare and the role they can play in advocating for preventative measures.

5.6. Capacity Building in Developing Nations

Developing nations may lack the resources and expertise to effectively combat biowarfare threats. International assistance and capacity-building programs can help these countries develop the infrastructure and expertise needed to prevent and respond to biowarfare incidents.

6.   The Role of the International Community

The international community has a collective responsibility to prevent and prosecute biowarfare crimes. Key stakeholders include:

6.1. United Nations

The United Nations plays a central role in coordinating international efforts to combat biowarfare. The UN Security Council can take action to address specific biowarfare incidents, while the General Assembly can facilitate discussions on strengthening the BWC and promoting international cooperation.

6.2. World Health Organization (WHO)

The WHO is instrumental in monitoring and responding to disease outbreaks, whether natural or intentional. Strengthening the WHO's capabilities for rapid response and investigation is crucial for addressing potential biowarfare incidents.

6.3. International Criminal Court (ICC)

The ICC has the authority to prosecute individuals for crimes against humanity, including biowarfare crimes. Expanding the ICC's jurisdiction to cover biowarfare-related offenses could serve as a powerful deterrent and mechanism for accountability.

Prosecuting biowarfare crimes is a complex and challenging endeavor. The global community must be proactive in preventing these crimes and holding perpetrators accountable when they occur. Strengthening the Biological Weapons Convention, enhancing international cooperation, promoting scientific collaboration, and raising public awareness are critical steps in addressing this grave threat to humanity.

As the world becomes more interconnected and the potential consequences of biowarfare more severe, the need for a comprehensive and coordinated response has never been greater. Only through a concerted effort by nations, international organizations, scientists, and legal experts can we hope to deter, detect, and prosecute biowarfare crimes effectively, ultimately safeguarding the health and security of people worldwide.

Societal Impact and Preparedness

Epidemics and pandemics have been a recurring feature of human history, shaping societies and economies in profound ways. From the Black Death in the 14th century to the Spanish flu in 1918 and more recently, the COVID-19 pandemic that began in 2019, these events have left an indelible mark on our collective memory. In this essay, we will delve into the societal impact of epidemics and pandemics throughout history, examining how societies have responded, and emphasizing the importance of preparedness in mitigating their effects.

I. Historical Context

To understand the societal impact of epidemics and pandemics, we must first examine their historical context. Throughout history, infectious diseases have periodically swept through human populations, causing significant morbidity and mortality. The Black Death, one of the deadliest pandemics in human history, killed an estimated 75-200 million people in Europe during the 14th century. This catastrophic event had profound societal consequences, including labor shortages, economic disruption, and social upheaval.

Similarly, the Spanish flu of 1918-1919 had a devastating impact on societies worldwide. With an estimated 50 million deaths worldwide, this pandemic disrupted daily life, overwhelmed healthcare systems, and created a deep sense of fear and uncertainty. It also exposed weaknesses in public health infrastructure and the need for better pandemic preparedness.

II. Societal Impact

Epidemics and pandemics have far-reaching societal impacts, affecting various aspects of human life:

1.   Healthcare Systems:
•   Overwhelmed healthcare systems: Epidemics and pandemics often strain healthcare infrastructure, leading to shortages of hospital beds, medical supplies, and personnel.
•   Re-prioritization of resources: Healthcare systems may need to divert resources from routine care to handle the surge in cases, affecting non-COVID-related health services.
2.   Economy:
•   Economic downturns: Epidemics and pandemics can trigger recessions as businesses close, trade declines, and unemployment rises.

- Supply chain disruptions: Global supply chains can be severely disrupted, leading to shortages of essential goods and increasing their prices.

3. Education:
- School closures: To mitigate the spread of disease, schools may be closed, disrupting students' education and exacerbating inequalities in access to learning.

4. Social Fabric:
- Isolation and mental health: Social distancing measures can lead to feelings of isolation and worsen mental health issues.
- Stigmatization: Fear and misinformation can lead to discrimination against affected communities or individuals.

5. Travel and Tourism:
- Travel restrictions: To contain the spread of the disease, governments often implement travel restrictions, affecting tourism and related industries.

6. Politics and Governance:
- Political response: Epidemics and pandemics can become political issues, with leaders facing challenges in managing public health crises effectively.
- Public trust: The response of governments and institutions can influence public trust and compliance with public health measures.

III. Preparedness

In light of the significant societal impact of epidemics and pandemics, preparedness is crucial. Effective preparedness involves a combination of strategies and actions at various levels:

1. Early Detection and Surveillance:
- Monitoring: Robust surveillance systems can detect outbreaks early, allowing for a swift response.
- International cooperation: Information sharing and collaboration between countries are essential to detect and contain global threats.

2. Healthcare Infrastructure:
- Healthcare capacity: Building and maintaining a resilient healthcare system with surge capacity is essential.
- Stockpiles: Maintaining stockpiles of medical supplies and equipment can ensure readiness.

3. Public Health Measures:
- Communication: Effective communication strategies, including clear public health messaging, are vital.
- Testing and contact tracing: Rapid testing and contact tracing help identify and isolate cases.

4. Research and Development:

•	Vaccine development: Investment in research and vaccine development can expedite responses to new pathogens.
•	Antiviral drugs: Developing effective antiviral drugs is essential to treat infected individuals.
5.	International Collaboration:
•	Global response: Epidemics and pandemics are global threats, necessitating international cooperation and coordination.
•	Preparedness frameworks: International organizations like the World Health Organization (WHO) play a crucial role in pandemic preparedness.
6.	Education and Training:
•	Healthcare workers: Training and equipping healthcare workers to respond to pandemics are essential.
•	Public awareness: Educating the public about infectious diseases and preventive measures is crucial.

IV. Lessons from COVID-19

The COVID-19 pandemic, which began in late 2019, offers numerous lessons on societal impact and preparedness. This global crisis highlighted the following key points:

1.	Importance of Scientific Advancements:
•	The rapid development of vaccines for COVID-19 demonstrated the value of scientific innovation in pandemic response.
2.	Global Interconnectedness:
•	The interconnectedness of the modern world facilitated the rapid spread of the virus, emphasizing the need for global cooperation.
3.	Role of Leadership:
•	Effective leadership at both national and international levels is critical in managing a pandemic.
4.	Resilience of Healthcare Systems:
•	Healthcare systems that were adequately prepared and adaptable fared better in responding to the crisis.
5.	Communication and Trust:
•	Clear and consistent communication from authorities was essential to building public trust and compliance with public health measures.
6.	Socioeconomic Disparities:
•	COVID-19 exposed and exacerbated existing socioeconomic disparities, with marginalized communities disproportionately affected.

V. Future Challenges

Looking ahead, several challenges must be addressed to enhance preparedness for future epidemics and pandemics:

1.   Vaccine Equity:
•   Ensuring equitable access to vaccines globally remains a pressing issue to prevent the emergence of new variants.
2.   Antimicrobial Resistance:
•   The rise of antimicrobial resistance poses a threat to our ability to treat infectious diseases effectively.
3.   Climate Change:
•   Climate change may increase the frequency of zoonotic diseases, necessitating a proactive approach to prevention.
4.   Misinformation:
•   The spread of misinformation and disinformation can hinder public health efforts during a crisis.
5.   Healthcare Infrastructure:
•   Strengthening healthcare infrastructure in low- and middle-income countries is crucial to global preparedness.

Epidemics and pandemics have played a significant role in shaping human history, with profound societal consequences. While we cannot predict when the next pandemic will occur, we can learn from past experiences and invest in preparedness measures. This includes early detection, robust healthcare infrastructure, global cooperation, and effective communication. The COVID-19 pandemic has underscored the importance of these factors and serves as a stark reminder of the need to be ready for future challenges in public health. By prioritizing preparedness, we can minimize the societal impact of epidemics and pandemics and better protect the well-being of our global community.

Psychological Effects

Epidemics and pandemics have been part of human history for centuries. These global health crises, often characterized by the rapid spread of infectious diseases, not only have a profound impact on physical health but also on the psychological well-being of individuals and communities. This article explores the various psychological effects of epidemics and pandemics, shedding light on the emotional, social, and mental health challenges that arise during these crises.

1.   Fear and Anxiety

One of the most immediate psychological effects of epidemics and pandemics is fear and anxiety. The uncertainty surrounding the transmission of the disease, its severity, and the potential consequences can lead to heightened levels of stress and worry. Fear of infection, illness, and death becomes pervasive, impacting individuals' mental health.

2.   Stigmatization and Discrimination

Epidemics often give rise to stigmatization and discrimination against those affected or perceived as carriers of the disease. This can lead to social isolation, ostracization, and negative mental health outcomes for both individuals and communities.

3.   Grief and Loss

Pandemics can result in significant loss of life, leaving behind a trail of grief and mourning. The collective experience of loss, along with the inability to hold traditional funeral ceremonies, can contribute to complicated grief and emotional distress.

4.   Loneliness and Social Isolation

Social distancing measures, such as lockdowns and quarantine, are commonly implemented during pandemics to slow the spread of the disease. While necessary from a public health standpoint, these measures can lead to social isolation, loneliness, and feelings of disconnectedness, all of which can have detrimental effects on mental health.

5.   Economic Stress

The economic fallout of pandemics, including job loss, business closures, and financial instability, can contribute to anxiety and depression. The fear of losing one's livelihood and the uncertainty of the future can be overwhelming.

6.   Psychological Impact on Healthcare Workers

Frontline healthcare workers are particularly vulnerable to the psychological effects of pandemics. They face extreme stress, burnout, and moral dilemmas, often leading to conditions like post-traumatic stress disorder (PTSD) and other mental health issues.

7.   Coping Mechanisms

Individuals employ various coping mechanisms during epidemics and pandemics. Some may resort to unhealthy behaviors like substance abuse or excessive consumption of media, while others may seek social support, engage in self-care practices, or turn to telehealth services for psychological support.

8.   Dissemination of Misinformation

The spread of misinformation and conspiracy theories during epidemics can exacerbate fear and anxiety. Efforts to combat false information are essential to maintaining trust and promoting mental well-being.

9.   Resilience and Adaptation

Despite the adverse psychological effects, many individuals and communities demonstrate resilience and adaptability during epidemics. They find innovative ways to cope with the challenges, support each other, and maintain a sense of hope.

10.   Mental Health Services and Support

Access to mental health services and support becomes crucial during epidemics and pandemics. Governments and organizations must prioritize the availability of mental health resources to address the growing demand. Telehealth services, crisis hotlines, and online support groups can play a vital role in providing assistance to individuals struggling with their mental health.

11.   Pre-existing Mental Health Conditions

Epidemics and pandemics can exacerbate pre-existing mental health conditions. Individuals with conditions like depression, anxiety, or OCD may experience heightened symptoms during these crises, making it essential for them to receive tailored support and treatment.

12.   Traumatic Experiences

For many, the experience of living through an epidemic or pandemic can be traumatic. Witnessing the suffering and loss of loved ones, being isolated from social support networks, or experiencing the illness personally can lead to long-lasting psychological trauma.

13.   The Impact on Children and Adolescents

Children and adolescents are not immune to the psychological effects of epidemics and pandemics. Disruption of routine, changes in schooling, and the stress experienced by their caregivers can have lasting consequences on their mental well-being.

14.   The Role of Social Media

The prevalence of social media during modern pandemics has both positive and negative implications. While it can help disseminate accurate information and connect individuals, it can also contribute to the spread of misinformation and fuel anxiety and panic.

15.   Long-term Effects

The psychological effects of epidemics and pandemics are not limited to the duration of the crisis. Long-term consequences, such as post-pandemic stress disorder (PPSD), may emerge, requiring ongoing mental health support and research.

16.   Lessons Learned

Epidemics and pandemics serve as stark reminders of the importance of preparedness and mental health awareness. Learning from past experiences, governments and healthcare systems can better address the psychological needs of their populations during future health crises.

17.   The Role of Resilience

Resilience, both at the individual and community levels, plays a significant role in mitigating the psychological effects of epidemics and pandemics. Strategies to enhance resilience should be incorporated into public health and disaster preparedness plans.

Epidemics and pandemics, while primarily public health crises, have far-reaching psychological effects on individuals and communities. The fear, anxiety, grief, and isolation experienced during these crises can have profound and long-lasting consequences on mental well-being. Recognizing and addressing these psychological effects is essential to promoting overall health and resilience in the face of future global health challenges.

As the world continues to grapple with the ongoing COVID-19 pandemic and prepares for potential future health crises, it is imperative that governments, healthcare systems, and communities prioritize mental health services and support. By doing so, we can mitigate the psychological impact of epidemics and pandemics and build a more resilient and mentally healthy society.

Community Resilience

The 21st century has witnessed several significant epidemics and pandemics, from the H1N1 influenza outbreak in 2009 to the Ebola crisis in West Africa in 2014-2016, and most notably, the COVID-19 pandemic that began in late 2019. These events have highlighted the critical importance of community resilience in responding to health crises. Community resilience refers to the ability of a community to withstand and recover from shocks, including epidemics and pandemics. This essay explores the concept of community resilience in the context of epidemics and pandemics, examining its components, challenges, and strategies to enhance it.

Understanding Community Resilience

Community resilience is a multifaceted concept that encompasses various dimensions, including social, economic, environmental, and health-related aspects. In the context of epidemics and pandemics, community resilience primarily focuses on the community's ability to effectively prepare for, respond to, and recover from health crises. It involves the following key components:

1.   Healthcare Infrastructure: A resilient community has a robust healthcare infrastructure, including hospitals, clinics, and healthcare professionals, capable of providing essential medical services during an epidemic or pandemic. The capacity to treat and isolate infected individuals is crucial in preventing the spread of diseases.
2.   Community Engagement: Resilience is built through active community engagement and participation. Community members must be informed, involved in decision-making, and educated about disease prevention measures. Trust between authorities and the community is vital for effective communication and cooperation.
3.   Economic Stability: Economic resilience involves maintaining economic stability during a health crisis. Communities with diverse economies and access to resources are better equipped to weather the economic impacts of pandemics, such as job loss and reduced economic activity.
4.   Social Cohesion: Strong social networks and cohesion are essential for community resilience. Communities with close-knit social ties are more likely to support vulnerable members, share information, and adhere to public health guidelines during epidemics.
5.   Adaptive Capacity: The ability to adapt and learn from past experiences is a hallmark of resilience. Communities that can adjust their strategies and policies based on lessons learned from previous epidemics are better prepared for future challenges.

Challenges to Community Resilience

Despite the importance of community resilience, several challenges can hinder its development and effectiveness in responding to epidemics and pandemics:

1.   Health Disparities: Socioeconomic and racial disparities in healthcare access can exacerbate the impact of diseases on vulnerable populations. Addressing these disparities is essential for building resilience.
2.   Misinformation: The spread of misinformation and disinformation can undermine community trust and hinder adherence to public health guidelines. Combatting misinformation requires effective communication strategies.
3.   Resource Constraints: Many communities, especially in low-income countries, lack the necessary resources to invest in healthcare infrastructure and preparedness measures. Resource constraints can limit a community's ability to respond effectively.
4.   Global Interconnectedness: In an increasingly interconnected world, diseases can spread rapidly across borders. Communities need to collaborate at local, national, and international levels to address global health threats.

Strategies to Enhance Community Resilience

To enhance community resilience in the face of epidemics and pandemics, various strategies can be implemented:

1.   Invest in Healthcare Infrastructure: Governments and organizations should invest in healthcare infrastructure, ensuring that hospitals and clinics have adequate resources, equipment, and trained personnel to handle disease outbreaks.
2.   Education and Communication: Public health campaigns and educational initiatives should be designed to inform and engage the community. Clear and accurate communication is vital in dispelling myths and misconceptions.
3.   Community-Based Interventions: Tailoring interventions to the specific needs and characteristics of each community can be highly effective. Local leaders and organizations can play a crucial role in designing and implementing these interventions.
4.   Resource Mobilization: Communities should work to mobilize resources from various sources, including government funding, philanthropy, and grants, to enhance their resilience.
5.   Collaboration and Coordination: Collaboration between different sectors, such as healthcare, government, and community organizations, is essential for a coordinated response. This includes international collaboration for addressing global health threats.
6.   Capacity Building: Training community members in essential skills, such as first aid and crisis management, can enhance a community's ability to respond effectively.
7.   Community Empowerment: Empowering community members to take an active role in decision-making and response efforts fosters a sense of ownership and responsibility.

Case Studies in Community Resilience

To better understand the concept of community resilience in the context of epidemics and pandemics, let's examine a few case studies:

1. Ebola Outbreak in West Africa (2014-2016)

The Ebola outbreak in West Africa exposed the vulnerabilities of the affected countries' healthcare systems. Communities in Guinea, Sierra Leone, and Liberia faced numerous challenges, including a lack of healthcare infrastructure, widespread misinformation, and mistrust of authorities. However, through international collaboration, community engagement, and capacity building, these countries were able to control the outbreak and build resilience for future health crises.

2. COVID-19 Response in New Zealand

New Zealand's response to the COVID-19 pandemic is often cited as a success story in community resilience. The government implemented a strict lockdown, engaged in clear and transparent communication, and relied on the cooperation of its citizens. This approach led to a swift containment of the virus and demonstrated the power of community resilience when supported by effective leadership.

3. Community-Led Responses in Low-Income Countries

In many low-income countries, where healthcare resources are limited, communities have taken the initiative to respond to epidemics. For example, during the Ebola outbreak in Sierra Leone, local organizations and community leaders played a crucial role in educating the population, providing care for the sick, and facilitating contact tracing. These community-led efforts demonstrated the resilience and adaptability of local populations.

Community resilience is a critical factor in responding to epidemics and pandemics. It involves various components, including healthcare infrastructure, community engagement, economic stability, social cohesion, and adaptive capacity. While challenges like health disparities, misinformation, and resource constraints exist, strategies such as investment in healthcare infrastructure, education and communication, and community-based interventions can enhance resilience.

The case studies of the Ebola outbreak in West Africa, New Zealand's COVID-19 response, and community-led efforts in low-income countries highlight the importance of community resilience in mitigating the impact of health crises. Building resilience is an ongoing process that requires collaboration, investment, and community empowerment. In a world where health threats are increasingly interconnected, prioritizing community resilience is essential to protect the well-being of populations and ensure a healthier future for all.

CONCLUSION

Biological Warfare, Epidemic, and Pandemic Outbreaks: A Looming Global Threat

In a world shaped by geopolitical tensions, rapid technological advancements, and interconnectedness, the specter of biological warfare, epidemic, and pandemic outbreaks looms large. This essay has explored the multifaceted nature of these threats, delving into the history, contemporary challenges, and potential future scenarios. The conclusion, therefore, serves as a synthesis of the key findings and a call to action.

Throughout history, biological warfare has existed as a dark undercurrent, with instances ranging from the use of plague-ridden corpses in medieval sieges to more recent allegations of state-sponsored bioterrorism. While the Biological Weapons Convention (BWC) of 1972 seeks to outlaw such practices, the ambiguous nature of biological research and dual-use technologies has made enforcement and verification challenging. The international community must reinforce its commitment to this treaty, foster greater transparency, and provide adequate resources for monitoring and compliance.

Epidemics and pandemics, on the other hand, have always been a part of human existence. However, the 21st century has witnessed an alarming increase in their frequency and scale. Factors such as urbanization, globalization, and climate change have accelerated the spread of infectious diseases. The COVID-19 pandemic serves as a stark reminder of our vulnerability. Thus, a holistic approach that combines robust healthcare systems, early warning mechanisms, and international collaboration is essential to mitigate these threats.

The intersection of biological warfare and pandemic outbreaks presents a particularly alarming scenario. The deliberate release of a deadly pathogen could lead to a catastrophic pandemic, causing widespread death and disruption. To counter this, nations must not only enhance their biological security measures but also cooperate internationally to prevent bioterrorism and biowarfare. This includes strengthening intelligence sharing, conducting joint exercises, and investing in countermeasures.

Furthermore, advances in biotechnology have raised the possibility of synthetic biology being used for malicious purposes. The democratization of these technologies means that non-state actors could potentially develop and release deadly pathogens. To address this, governments and international bodies must implement stringent regulations on gene-editing and synthetic biology research, while also promoting responsible innovation.

The importance of public health preparedness cannot be overstated. Investing in research, surveillance, and vaccine development is crucial. Additionally, healthcare systems must be flexible and resilient, capable of responding swiftly to emerging threats. Public education and awareness campaigns should also be prioritized to ensure that individuals are informed and empowered to protect themselves and their communities.

International cooperation is paramount in addressing these complex challenges. Global health security should be elevated to the same level of importance as national security. The World Health Organization (WHO) must be adequately funded and empowered to coordinate responses to epidemics and pandemics. Bilateral and multilateral partnerships, including information sharing and resource allocation, are essential to ensure a coordinated global response.

The role of technology in combating biological threats cannot be ignored. Artificial intelligence (AI) and big data analytics can assist in tracking disease outbreaks, predicting their spread, and optimizing resource allocation. Furthermore, the development of rapid diagnostic tools and vaccine platforms can significantly reduce response times during emergencies.

Ethical considerations also play a significant role in this landscape. The balance between individual privacy and public health surveillance is a delicate one. Striking the right balance requires ongoing discourse, legislation, and oversight to protect civil liberties while safeguarding public health.

In conclusion, the convergence of biological warfare, epidemic, and pandemic outbreaks represents a multifaceted and ever-evolving global threat. History has shown that these threats are not hypothetical; they are real and can have devastating consequences. Therefore, proactive measures are imperative.

The international community must prioritize the strengthening and enforcement of the Biological Weapons Convention. Robust biological security measures, responsible innovation, and stringent regulations on gene-editing and synthetic biology are needed to prevent bioterrorism and biowarfare. Investments in public health preparedness, research, and healthcare infrastructure must be made to mitigate the impact of epidemics and pandemics.

Furthermore, international cooperation, through organizations like the WHO, must be enhanced to facilitate a coordinated response to global health crises. Technology, including AI and big data analytics, should be harnessed to improve disease surveillance and response times. Ethical considerations should guide the use of technology and the balance between privacy and public health.

The world stands at a crossroads. The choices we make today will determine our ability to confront and mitigate the complex challenges of biological warfare, epidemic, and pandemic outbreaks. The lessons of history and the urgency of the present demand nothing less than a concerted, global effort to secure the health and safety of humanity. The time for action is now.

Looking Ahead: The Future of Biological Warfare and Pandemics

Biological Warfare and Pandemics: A Glimpse into the Future

The world has experienced several pandemics throughout history, from the Spanish flu of 1918 to the more recent COVID-19 pandemic that began in 2019. These outbreaks have not only taken a toll on human lives but have also exposed vulnerabilities in our global healthcare and preparedness systems. As we move forward into an increasingly interconnected and technologically advanced world, it's crucial to examine the potential future of biological warfare and pandemics. In this exploration, we will consider the evolving landscape of biological threats, the role of technology, and the measures needed to safeguard humanity.

Part 1: The Evolution of Biological Warfare

1.1 Historical Perspective

Biological warfare, the use of disease-causing microorganisms as weapons, has a long and dark history. From the intentional distribution of smallpox-infected blankets by European colonists to Native Americans in the 18th century to Japan's Unit 731 experiments during World War II, humans have explored the deadly potential of biological agents. However, as we look ahead, the face of biological warfare is poised to change dramatically.

1.2 Modern Advancements

The 21st century has ushered in a new era of biological warfare. Advances in biotechnology and synthetic biology have made it easier than ever to manipulate microorganisms, modify their virulence, and engineer novel pathogens. CRISPR gene-editing technology, for instance, allows precise modifications to the genetic makeup of bacteria and viruses. This raises concerns about the potential creation of designer pathogens with increased transmissibility and lethality.

1.3 State Actors and Non-State Threats

Traditionally, nation-states have been the primary actors in biological warfare. However, as biotechnology becomes more accessible, non-state actors, including terrorist groups and individuals, could pose significant threats. DIY biology labs and the availability of genetic information online make it increasingly feasible for motivated individuals to embark on dangerous bioweapon projects.

Part 2: The Changing Nature of Pandemics

2.1 Zoonotic Spillover

Many pandemics originate from the transmission of pathogens from animals to humans, known as zoonotic spillover. Deforestation, urbanization, and the global wildlife trade create environments where such spillover events are more likely to occur. Looking ahead, we must address the root causes of zoonotic diseases to prevent future pandemics.

2.2 Antimicrobial Resistance

The misuse of antibiotics and antimicrobial agents has led to the rise of antimicrobial resistance (AMR). This phenomenon threatens to render our most potent weapons against infectious diseases ineffective. As we face the future, tackling AMR is a paramount challenge in pandemic preparedness.

2.3 The Role of Climate Change

Climate change influences the distribution and prevalence of infectious diseases. Rising temperatures, altered precipitation patterns, and habitat disruptions can expand the range of disease vectors and impact the dynamics of pandemics. Adaptation and mitigation strategies must be integrated into pandemic planning.

Part 3: Technology's Influence on Biological Warfare and Pandemics

3.1 Surveillance and Early Detection

Advances in surveillance technologies, including AI and machine learning, have improved our ability to detect outbreaks early. Predictive modeling and real-time data analysis allow for more effective responses, potentially averting large-scale pandemics.

3.2 Vaccine Development and Distribution

The development of vaccines has accelerated with the help of cutting-edge technologies like messenger RNA (mRNA) vaccines, as seen in the rapid creation of COVID-19 vaccines. Innovative distribution methods, such as drone delivery and mRNA vaccine platforms, promise to revolutionize pandemic response.

3.3 Biosecurity and Dual-Use Research

Striking a balance between scientific research and biosecurity is vital. Dual-use research, which can have both civilian and military applications, requires strict oversight. Enhanced biosecurity measures and international cooperation are essential to prevent the misuse of research.

Part 4: Preparing for the Future

4.1 Strengthening Global Health Infrastructure

The COVID-19 pandemic exposed critical weaknesses in global healthcare systems. Investments in healthcare infrastructure, including robust supply chains, well-equipped hospitals, and a trained workforce, are crucial for future preparedness.

4.2 International Collaboration

Pandemics and biological warfare threats transcend borders. International cooperation and information sharing are essential to identify and respond to emerging threats swiftly. Mechanisms like the World Health Organization (WHO) must be strengthened to fulfill their roles effectively.

4.3 Ethical Considerations

As we face the future of biological warfare and pandemics, ethical dilemmas will abound. Balancing individual privacy with public health surveillance, regulating potentially dangerous research, and ensuring equitable access to treatments and vaccines are ethical challenges that demand careful consideration.

The future of biological warfare and pandemics is marked by both promise and peril. Technology offers unprecedented tools for surveillance, vaccine development, and disease prevention, yet it also opens the door to new forms of bioterrorism. To safeguard humanity, we must address the evolving landscape of biological threats, prioritize global health infrastructure, and engage in international cooperation. As we look ahead, the lessons learned from past pandemics and the ethical principles we uphold will be our guiding lights in an uncertain future.

The Role of Science and Policy

Epidemics and pandemics are recurring threats to global public health, causing widespread illness, death, and economic disruptions. The effective management and control of these outbreaks depend on a complex interplay between science and policy. In this comprehensive essay, we will explore the critical roles that science and policy play in addressing epidemic and pandemic outbreaks, emphasizing their interdependence, challenges, and lessons learned.

Section 1: Understanding Epidemics and Pandemics

1.1 Definitions and Distinctions

Epidemics and pandemics are distinct in terms of scale and impact. An epidemic is a sudden increase in the number of cases of a particular disease in a defined geographical area, whereas a pandemic occurs when an epidemic becomes global, affecting multiple countries or continents.

1.2 The Role of Epidemiology

Epidemiology, the study of the distribution and determinants of diseases in populations, is fundamental in understanding outbreaks. Epidemiologists use data and statistical methods to identify patterns, risk factors, and transmission dynamics of infectious diseases.

Section 2: The Scientific Response

2.1 Early Detection and Surveillance

Timely detection is crucial in managing outbreaks. Scientific tools such as molecular diagnostics, serological testing, and data analytics have significantly improved our ability to detect and track the spread of infectious agents.

2.2 Vaccine Development and Therapeutics

Science plays a pivotal role in developing vaccines and treatments. Advancements in biotechnology, genomics, and immunology have accelerated the development of vaccines for emerging diseases like COVID-19.

2.3 Modeling and Predictive Analytics

Mathematical models help policymakers understand the potential trajectory of an outbreak. Models take into account variables such as transmission rates, population density, and public health interventions, assisting in decision-making.

Section 3: The Interplay with Policy

3.1 Policy Frameworks for Epidemics and Pandemics

Effective policies are essential to control outbreaks. Preparedness plans, containment strategies, and international cooperation frameworks (e.g., the International Health Regulations) guide countries in responding to epidemics and pandemics.

3.2 Decision-Making Processes

Science informs policy decisions, but policymakers must navigate uncertainty and balance public health with economic and social considerations. Ethical and equity issues also shape policy choices.

3.3 Public Communication and Risk Communication

Transparent and effective communication is crucial during outbreaks. Public health officials must convey scientific information accurately, addressing misinformation and fostering public trust.

Section 4: Challenges and Lessons Learned

4.1 Challenges in the Scientific Sphere

- Data quality and availability can hinder early detection and modeling accuracy.
- Rapid mutations in pathogens pose challenges to vaccine development.
- Science must adapt to emerging diseases and evolving threats.

4.2 Policy Challenges

- Balancing individual freedoms with public health measures can lead to controversy.
- International coordination and cooperation are often lacking during pandemics.
- The economic and social consequences of containment measures require careful consideration.

4.3 Lessons Learned from Past Outbreaks

Historical outbreaks like the Spanish flu, HIV /AIDS, and Ebola have provided valuable lessons for both science and policy:

- The importance of preparedness: Prior planning and investment in public health infrastructure are critical. Countries with robust healthcare systems and emergency response plans have fared better in managing outbreaks.
- The need for global cooperation: Infectious diseases do not respect borders. International collaboration and information sharing are essential to control pandemics effectively. Initiatives like COVAX for COVID-19 vaccine distribution highlight the importance of solidarity.
- Trust and communication: Building and maintaining trust between the scientific community, policymakers, and the public is crucial. Open, clear, and consistent communication helps reduce fear and misinformation.

Section 5: Case Study - COVID-19 Pandemic

5.1 The Emergence of SARS-CoV-2

The COVID-19 pandemic serves as a contemporary example of the interplay between science and policy. The emergence of the novel coronavirus posed a global threat, requiring rapid scientific response and policy action.

5.2 Scientific Contributions

- The identification of the virus and its genomic sequencing.
- Development of diagnostic tests.
- Collaborative efforts in vaccine development, leading to the creation of multiple effective vaccines in record time.

5.3 Policy Responses

- Widespread lockdowns, social distancing, and mask mandates.
- Accelerated regulatory approvals for vaccines and treatments.
- Financial support for healthcare systems and individuals affected by the economic downturn.

Section 6: The Path Forward

6.1 Strengthening Global Health Systems

Investment in healthcare infrastructure, workforce training, and supply chain resilience is essential for future preparedness.

6.2 Advancing Scientific Tools and Research

Continued research in virology, genomics, and disease modeling will enhance our ability to respond swiftly to emerging threats.

6.3 Policy Reforms and International Collaboration

Reforming policies to streamline decision-making during crises and fostering international cooperation are imperative for global health security.

The role of science and policy in epidemic and pandemic outbreaks is intertwined and vital. Scientific advancements provide the knowledge needed to combat infectious diseases, while policies guide the implementation of preventive measures and treatments. The challenges posed by outbreaks are significant, but history has shown that humanity can adapt, learn, and evolve in response to these threats. By embracing the lessons of the past and committing to cooperation, we can better protect global health in an interconnected world. The COVID-19 pandemic serves as a stark reminder of the importance of this dynamic relationship, urging us to remain vigilant and prepared for the challenges that lie ahead.

Appendices A:

Glossary of Terms

- Biological Warfare: The use of biological agents, such as bacteria, viruses, or toxins, as weapons to harm or kill humans, animals, or plants.
- Epidemic: The rapid spread of a disease to a large number of people in a specific geographic area.
- Pandemic: An epidemic that has spread over multiple countries or continents, affecting a significant portion of the global population.
- Biological Agent: Microorganisms (e.g., bacteria, viruses), toxins, or other biological substances used in biological warfare.
- Containment: Strategies and measures taken to prevent the spread of a disease outbreak.
- Quarantine: The isolation of individuals who may have been exposed to a contagious disease to prevent its spread.
- Vaccination: The process of administering vaccines to stimulate immunity against specific diseases.
- Zoonotic Disease: Diseases that can be transmitted from animals to humans, often a concern in biological warfare.
- Bioterrorism: Deliberate use of biological agents or toxins to cause harm or fear among a population.
- PPE (Personal Protective Equipment): Equipment such as masks, gloves, and suits used to protect against biological hazards.

Appendices B: ADDITIONAL RESOURCES

"Biological Warfare: A Historical Perspective" by Mark Wheelis, Lajos Rózsa, and Malcolm Dando (Annual Review of Microbiology, 2006).

"Biological Weapons: Recognizing, Understanding, and Responding to the Threat" by Barry R. Schneider and Jim A. Davis (Johns Hopkins University Press, 2017).

"The Invisible Enemy: A Natural History of Viruses" by Dorothy H. Crawford (Oxford University Press, 2001).

"The Next Pandemic: On the Front Lines Against Humankind's Gravest Dangers" by Ali S. Khan (PublicAffairs, 2016).

"Pandemics: A Very Short Introduction" by Christian W. McMillen (Oxford University Press, 2016).

INDEXES

Index on Biological Warfare:

1.   Definition of Biological Warfare: An overview of what biological warfare is, including its history and methods.
2.   Biological Agents: Information on various biological agents used in warfare, such as bacteria, viruses, and toxins.
3.   Historical Examples: A look at significant historical incidents involving biological warfare, like anthrax attacks and bioterrorism.
4.   Treaties and Conventions: An overview of international agreements and conventions that prohibit the use of biological weapons.
5.   Current Threats: Discussion of contemporary concerns and potential threats related to biological warfare.
6.   Countermeasures: Information on efforts to prevent and respond to biological warfare, including biosecurity measures and preparedness.

Introduction on Epidemic and Pandemic Outbreaks:

Epidemics and pandemics are global health crises characterized by the rapid spread of infectious diseases. Here's an introduction to these topics:

Epidemics:

Epidemics are outbreaks of infectious diseases that occur within a specific geographic area or community. They typically affect a larger number of people than expected and may overwhelm local healthcare systems. Key points include:

•   Causes: Epidemics can be caused by various factors, including new pathogens, changes in host behavior, or breakdowns in public health measures.
•   Impact: Epidemics can result in significant illness, death, and economic disruption, but their scope is usually limited to a specific region.

Pandemics:

Pandemics are global epidemics, characterized by the worldwide spread of a new infectious disease. They have the potential to affect a large portion of the global population. Key points include:

- Global Impact: Pandemics can affect multiple countries and continents, leading to widespread illness and societal disruption.
- Examples: Historical pandemics include the 1918 influenza pandemic (Spanish flu) and the more recent COVID-19 pandemic.

9 798861 605984